Emerald

1

© Straightforward Publishing 2016

British Cataloguing in Publication data. A catalogue record is available for this book from the British Library.

ISBN
978-1-84716-662-3

Printed in the United Kingdom by 4edge www.4edge.co.uk

Cover Design by Bookworks Islington

Contents

Introduction

****

Introduction

In the Times Newspaper, Thursday 28th July 2016, the main headline was:

'Scientists create the first drug to halt Alzheimer's'.

Reading further into the report, as it is always necessary to do, without a doubt this comes as a very welcome development indeed. The treatment consists of a pill, taken twice a day which halts mental decline for as much as 18 months in some patients. The research came from McGill university and was presented to the Alzheimer's Association annual conference in Toronto, Canada.

Another report from the University of Manchester states that Mefenamic acid, a drug used for the prevention of period pains, has been found, after tests on mice, to reverse Alzheimer's. However, once again, it is necessary to be cautious, because what works on mice may not work on human beings. The tests will now be extended to people.

Many of us who welcomed these findings will have had some dealings with the onset of dementia, either directly through family or through the experience of friends, or through the workplace if we are involved in the care industry. Often, we will have seen the tragic consequences of the effects of dementia, be it

Alzheimer's or one of the other manifestations of the condition, which are outlined in chapter 2.

My mothers twin sister, 88 years of age sufferers with Alzheimer's and my mother feels helpless and is heartbroken that nothing can be done to help at this late point. The experience of my mother, and also people I know who have been directly involved has prompted me to write this book, in the hope that the information contained within can possibly help people involved alleviate the condition through early intervention and also highlight the existence of support groups and national organisations which can provide invaluable advice and help along the journey.

In 2014, one of the major national organisations, The Alzheimer's Society, produced a set of statistics which revealed the true extent of dementia in the United Kingdom. The following are some of the findings, which make harrowing reading:

- By 2015 there will be 850,000 people with dementia in the UK. (proven now in 2016)
- There are 40,000 younger people with dementia in the UK.
- There are 25,000 people with dementia from black and minority ethnic groups in the UK.
- There will be 2 million people with dementia in the UK by 2025.
- Two thirds of people with dementia are women.

- The proportion of people with dementia doubles for every five-year age group.
- One in six people aged 80 and over have dementia.
- 60,000 deaths a year are directly attributable to dementia.
- Delaying the onset of dementia by five years would reduce deaths directly attributable to dementia by 30,000 a year.
- The financial cost of dementia to the UK is £26 billion per annum.
- There are 670,000 carers of people with dementia in the UK.
- Family carers of people with dementia save the UK £11 billion a year.
- 80 per cent of people living in care homes have a form of dementia or severe memory problems.
- Two thirds of people with dementia live in the community while one third live in a care home.
- Only 44% of people with dementia in England, Wales and Northern Ireland receive a diagnosis

The Impact of dementia
Dementia costs the UK £26.3 Billion a year, which is enough to pay the annual energy bill of every household in the country.

Too many people with dementia aren't living as well as they could
- 61% felt anxious or depressed recently
- 40% felt lonely recently.

- 52% don't feel they get enough support from the government.
- 34% don't feel part of their community.
- 28% aren't able to make decisions about how they spend their time.
- 18% aren't living well with dementia.

Services need to reflect the needs of individuals.
1 out of 20 people living with dementia are under the age of 65. 7 out of 10 people are living with another medical condition or disability as well as dementia.

The above figures are produced from a report made by the Alzheimer's society in 2014. www.alzheimers.org.uk

Government policy on dementia
In the light of the above figures, and an acknowledgement of dementia as a growing crisis, the government has produced a policy aimed at tackling the problem, as summarised below.

DOH Policy

The Department of Health wants every person with dementia, and their carers and families, – from all backgrounds, walks of life and in all parts of the country – to receive high quality, compassionate care from diagnosis through to end of life care. This applies to all care settings, whether home, hospital or care home.

People with dementia have told us what is important to them. They want a society where they are able to say:

- I have personal choice and control over the decisions that affect me.
- I know that services are designed around me, my needs and my carer's needs.
- I have support that helps me live my life.
- I have the knowledge to get what I need.
- I live in an enabling and supportive environment where I feel valued and understood.
- I have a sense of belonging and of being a valued part of family, community and civic life.
- I am confident my end of life wishes will be respected. I can expect a good death.
- I know that there is research going on which will deliver a better life for people with dementia, and I know how I can contribute to it.

The Department of Health wants:

- the best services and innovation currently delivered in some parts of the country to be delivered everywhere
- a society where kindness, care and dignity take precedence over structures or systems
- the wellbeing and quality of life of people with dementia and their family/carers to be uppermost in the minds of those commissioning and providing services

- greater recognition that everyone with dementia is an individual with specific needs
- people with dementia and their carers to be fully involved in decisions, not only about their own care, but also in the commissioning and development of services

This vision is set out in the Prime Minister's challenge on dementia 2020. This is an aspirational document, which builds on the achievements of the Prime Minister's challenge on dementia 2012-2015, and aims to identify what needs to be done to make sure that dementia care, support, awareness and research are transformed by 2020. It also outlines the progress that has been made so far on the main elements of the original 3-year dementia challenge – health and care, dementia friendly communities and research.

The 2020 challenge document doesn't mandate actions, or make spending commitments. What happens in the years to 2020 will be determined by the next government in the context of the Spending Review. The full policy can be viewed by going to https://www.gov.uk/government/policies/dementia.

In the light of the ongoing crisis surrounding the growth of dementia, it is obvious that more and more time and effort is being spent on looking for cures, in the main trying to prevent the onset of the condition. As we will see, many organisations, such as the NHS, Social Services and national groups such as The Alzheimer's Society and Dementia Action Alliance are continuously working with dementia sufferers and their families. The useful resources section at the back of the book outlines numerous organisations, most of them voluntary which provide invaluable help and support.

In the book, the following areas are discussed:

o   Chapter 1 covers the nature of dementia and also the various manifestations of the condition.
o   Chapter 2 covers the treatment and prevention of dementia
o   Chapter 3 covers the experience of living with Dementia and Alzheimer's from the vantage point of the actual sufferer and also their families. Practical advice on the many areas affecting people is outlined.
o   Chapter 4 deals with legal and financial matters
o   Chapter 5 covers wider support networks, such as the NHS, Social Services and other groups which operate nationally and locally.
o   Chapter 6 covers local authority/social services assessments and care plans
o   Chapter 7 covers welfare benefits available for dementia sufferers and their carers
o   Chapter 8 covers the role of diet and exercise in helping dementia sufferers.

There is a comprehensive resource section at the back of the book which should provide invaluable advice and guidance. In addition, appendix 1 contains valuable information about current benefit rates.

Chapter 1

The Nature of Dementia

What is dementia?

Dementia is caused by diseases of the brain, the most common form of which is Alzheimer's disease.

Dementia is the loss of cognitive functioning, thinking, remembering, and reasoning and also behavioral abilities to such an extent that it interferes with a person's daily life and activities. Dementia ranges in severity from the mildest stage, when it is just beginning to affect a person's functioning, to the most severe stage, when the person must depend completely on others for basic activities of daily living.

The causes of dementia can vary, depending on the types of brain changes that may be taking place. As mentioned above, the most commonly known form is Alzheimer's disease. Other dementias include Lewy body dementia, Frontotemporal disorders, Vascular dementia, Creutzfeldt-Kakob disease, Huntington's disease, Wernicke-Korsakoff Syndrome, and normal pressure hydrocephalus. In addition, Parkinson's disease can result in progressive dementia similar to Alzheimers. It is common for people to have mixed dementia—a combination of two or more disorders, at least one of which is dementia. For example, some people have both Alzheimer's disease and vascular dementia.

Other conditions that may cause memory loss or dementia include:

- medication side effects
- chronic alcoholism
- tumors or infections in the brain
- blood clots in the brain
- vitamin B12 deficiency
- some thyroid, kidney, or liver disorders
- stroke
- Parkinson's disease
- sleep disturbances

Some of these conditions may be treatable and possibly reversible. They can be serious and should be treated by a doctor as soon as possible. Emotional problems, such as stress, anxiety, or depression, can make a person more forgetful and can be mistaken for dementia. For instance, someone who has recently retired or who is coping with the death of a spouse may feel sad, lonely, worried, or bored. Trying to deal with these life changes leaves some people confused or forgetful. The emotional problems can be eased by supportive friends and family, but if these feelings last for a long time, it is important to get help from a doctor or counselor.

Alzheimer's disease is the most common cause of dementia amongst older adults.

What is Alzheimer's disease?

A few decades ago, only a few medical specialists would have heard of Alzheimer's disease. "Senility" was considered inevitable for anyone who lived long enough. But as understanding of the brain has grown, science has been able to identify and differentiate many causes of dementia. Alzheimer's is the most common type of dementia, but other brain disorders can and do frequently cause dementia.

Alzheimer's disease is an irreversible, progressive brain disorder that slowly destroys memory and thinking skills and, eventually, the ability to carry out the simplest tasks. In most people with Alzheimer's, symptoms first appear in their mid-60s. The disease is named after Dr. Alois Alzheimer. In 1906, Dr. Alzheimer noticed changes in the brain tissue of a woman who had died of an unusual mental illness. Her symptoms included memory loss, language problems, and unpredictable behavior. After she died, he examined her brain and found many abnormal clumps (now called Amyloid plaques) and tangled bundles of fibers (now called neurofibrillary, or Tau tangles).

These plaques and tangles in the brain are still considered some of the main features of Alzheimer's disease. Another feature is the loss of connections between nerve cells (neurons) in the brain. Neurons transmit messages between different parts of the brain, and from the brain to muscles and organs in the body. Although treatment can help manage symptoms in some people, currently there is no cure for this devastating disease.

What happens to the brain in Alzheimer's disease?

Scientists continue to unravel the complex brain changes involved in the onset and progression of Alzheimer's disease. It seems likely that damage to the brain starts a decade or more before memory and other cognitive problems become evident. During this pre-clinical stage of Alzheimer's disease, people seem to be symptom-free, but toxic changes are taking place in the brain. Abnormal deposits of proteins form amyloid plaques and tau tangles throughout the brain, and once-healthy neurons stop functioning, lose connections with other neurons, and die.

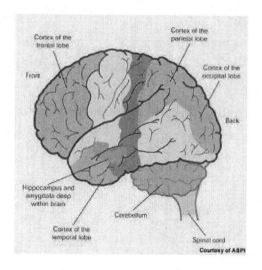

Alzheimer's Brain

The damage initially appears to take place in the hippocampus, the part of the brain essential in forming memories. As more neurons die, additional parts of the brain are affected. By the final stage of Alzheimer's, damage is widespread, and brain tissue has shrunk significantly.

How long can a person live with Alzheimer's disease?

Alzheimer's is a slow disease that progresses in three stages—an early, pre-clinical stage with no symptoms, a middle stage of mild cognitive impairment, and a final stage of Alzheimer's dementia. The time from diagnosis to death varies—as little as 3 or 4 years if the person is older than 80 when diagnosed to as long as 10 or more years if the person is younger.

Other types of dementia-Vascular Dementia

Vascular dementia is also known as "Multi-infarct dementia" or "Post-stroke dementia" and is the second most common cause of dementia.

Main symptoms:

- Memory loss
- Impaired judgment
- Decreased ability to plan
- Loss of motivation

Cause: Bleeding within the brain from a stroke causes brain damage.

Treatments or therapies: Vascular dementia cannot be cured, but people who have the ailment are treated to prevent further brain injury from the underlying cause of the ailment. Like

Alzheimer's disease, numerous medication and therapies may be used to help manage the symptoms.

Lewy Body Dementia

Lewy body dementia is the third most common cause of dementia, and is also called "cortical Lewy body disease" or "diffuse Lewy body disease."

Main symptoms:

- Sleep problems
- Memory loss
- Hallucinations
- Frequent swings in alertness

Cause: Lewy bodies, abnormal proteins that somehow appear in nerve cells and impair functioning.

Treatments or therapies: There is no known treatment to reverse Lewy body dementia or address its underlying cellular cause, but as with Alzheimer's and other main types of dementia, a wide array of therapies and treatment are used to improve the patient's quality of life and alleviate symptoms.

Frontotemporal Dementia

Frontotemporal dementia is fairly rare, but believed to be the fourth most common type of dementia. Unlike the types of dementia discussed previously, frontotemporal dementia is marked more by behavioral and emotional changes than by cognitive impairment. In fact, memory is preserved in people with frontotemporal dementia.

Main symptoms:
- Decreased inhibition (frequently leading to inappropriate behavior)
- Apathy and loss of motivation-Decreased empathy
- Repetitive or compulsive behaviors
- Anxiety and depression

Cause: Frontotemporal dementia occurs when the frontal or temporal lobes of the brain are damaged or shrink.

Treatments or therapies: Frontotemporal dementia cannot be cured or reversed, but doctors will use medicines to treat uncomfortable or problematic symptoms.

Creutzfeldt-Jakob disease

CJD is the most common human form of a rare, fatal brain disorder affecting people and certain other mammals. Variant CJD (Mad Cow Disease) occurs in cattle, and has been transmitted to people under certain circumstances. The main symptom of CJD is a rapidly fading disorder that impairs memory and co-ordination and causes behaviour changes

Normal pressure hydrocephalus

This is caused by a build up of fluid on the brain and can sometimes be corrected by draining off the fluid. Symptoms include difficulty in walking, memory loss and inability to control urination.

Huntington's disease

Huntington's disease is a progressive brain disorder caused by a single defective gene. The symptoms include abnormal involuntary movements, a severe decline in thinking and reasoning skills, irritability, depression and mood changes.

Wernicke-Korsakoff Syndrome

Korsakoff syndrome is a chronic memory disorder caused by severe deficiency if thiamine (vitamin B-1). The most common cause is alcohol abuse. Memory problems become strikingly severe and social skills can remain relatively unaffected.

Parkinson's disease

As Parkinson's progresses, it often results in a progressive dementia similar to dementia with Lewy bodies or Alzheimer's.

The root of Parkinson's lies within the brain. Scientific research has determined that bodily movements are regulated by an area of the brain called the basal ganglia, whose cells require a proper balance of substances known as d*opamine* and *acetylcholine*, both involved in the transmission of nerve impulses. With Parkinson's, cells that produce dopamine begin to degenerate. When this happens, the insufficient dopamine disturbs the balance between dopamine and other transmitters, such as acetylcholine. Therefore, dopamine can be seen as a chemical messenger responsible for transmitting signals between the substantia nigra and the next 'relay station' of the brain, which is the corpus striatum, to produce smooth, purposeful muscle activity. Loss of dopamine causes the nerve cells of the striatum to fire out of control, leaving the person unable to direct or control their movements in a normal manner.

The exact cause of this cell death or impairment is unknown. However, scientists have made advances in this area and one theory holds that free radicals, unstable and potentially damaging molecules generated by normal chemical reactions in the body, may contribute to nerve cell death that leads to Parkinson's.

Young onset dementia

What is young onset dementia?
Dementia is considered to be 'young onset' when it affects people under 65 years of age. It is also referred to as 'early onset' or 'working age' dementia. However, although the classification is under 65, this is an arbitary age distinction which is considered to be too rigid and which is becoming less relevant as increasingly services are realigned to focus on the actual person and the impact of the condition, not the age.

Dementias that affect younger people can be rare and difficult to recognise. People can also be very reluctant to accept there is anything wrong when they are otherwise fit and well, and they may put off visiting their doctor.

The impact for younger people and their families
Although younger people experience similar symptoms to older people with dementia, the impact on their lives is significantly different and problematic in different ways. Younger people are more likely to still be working when they are diagnosed. Many will have significant financial commitments such as a mortgage. They often have children to care for and dependent parents too.

Therefore, as the problem advances, specialised advice will be needed.

The Alzheimer's Society and also the NHS can provide a wide range of advice and support to those affected by dementia at an earlier age.

In Chapter 2, we will look at methods of treating dementia, including medication. As we will see, there are a number of medications that can be used, also psychological treatments. However, equally effective is prevention in the first place through modification in lifestyle.

****

Chapter 2

Treating Dementia and Preventing Dementia

How is dementia treated?
In the main, although most types of dementia cannot be treated, and will slowly and gradually cause severe problems for the sufferer and their family and friends, there are a few exceptions such as dementia caused by vitamin deficiency and also thyroid hormone deficiency, which can be treated by supplements. Some causes, as mentioned in Chapter 1, can be treated surgically, such as fluid on the brain (hydrocephalus) brain tumours and head injuries.

As we will discuss later, for types of dementia that involve degeneration of nerve and brain tissue, action can be taken to prevent further damage by reducing dementia risk factors such as managing high blood pressure, stopping smoking, high cholesterol and managing diabetes.

For dementia that cannot be cured, there are some types of medicine on the market that may prevent symptoms getting worse, at least for a period of time. As was pointed out in the introduction, scientists are making advances and claim to have created the first drug to cure Alzheimer's.

Medicines to treat dementia

There are a number of medicines which have been shown to be effective in treating mild, moderate and severe dementia. However, not everyone will benefit from these. The most effective treatment is the early prevention and involves changes in lifestyle, as discussed further on in this chapter.

The following are the medicines most widely prescribed by doctor's when treating dementia.

Aricept (donepezil) and acetylcholinesterase inhibitors

Acetylcholinesterase inhibitors such as galantamine and rivastigmine, are used to treat mild to moderate Alzheimer's disease. They are also used to treat dementia with Lewy bodies and can be quite effective, particularly at treating hallucinations. As with all medication, there can be side effects, such as nausea and vomiting but they are short lived. Another side effect can be the slowing down of the heartbeat, so doctors will usually advise an electrocardiogram (ECG) before treatment.

Memantine hydrochloride

Memantine is a medicine that works by blocking the effects of a chemical in the brain. This is usually prescribed to those with severe Alzheimer's disease but can also be given to those with moderate symptoms.

Anti-psychotics

Anti-psychotics are used to treat people who's behaviour is disruptive, for example they become aggressive or agitated, which is a common symptom of Alzheimer's, particularly in the later stages. However, they are normally used for a short period of time because of the potential side effects, such as cardiovascular problems and drowsiness. There is a debate as to whether these types of drugs should be used at all as they can worsen the condition. Before anti-psychotic drugs are used, the doctor will usually discuss the side effects, or potential side effects with family or friends.

Anti-depressants

Dementia sufferers will usually suffer from depression and depression will normally result in a worsening of the memory and the ability to function. It is for this reason that anti-depressants are often prescribed.

Psychological treatments

It is well known that psychological treatments do not slow down the progression of dementia but they can help with the symptoms. There are a number of recommended therapies.

Cognitive stimulation and reality orientation therapy

Cognitive stimulation, as the name suggests, will involve exercises and taking part in activities which are designed to improve the memory and promote language and other skills.

Reality orientation therapy helps to reduce feelings of disorientation that arise with dementia, along with memory loss and confusion. It is hoped that self-esteem will be improved using this approach.

The National Institute for Health and Care Excellence (NICE) recommends the use of cognitive therapy to help people with mild or moderate dementia.

Validation therapy and behavioural therapy

Validation therapy focuses on dementia from an emotional perspective and is based on the principle that even the most confused behaviour has some meaning to the person involved, whilst behavioural therapy tries to find reasons for difficult behaviour. An example of validation therapy might be that if a person becomes agitated at a certain point in time because they believe a relative is visiting, telling them that their relatives are not coming could worsen the situation. Validation therapy involves talking to the person about the issue and gently steering the conversation away and in another direction. In theory, this should reduce their distress.

An example of behavioural therapy might be in a situation where a person is given to wandering aimlessly. They can be encouraged to take part in physical activity to focus their energy.

Preventing dementia

As we discussed earlier, medication for dementia, or at least the most severe forms of dementia is limited. As important as medication, which can quite often only delay or suppress symptoms, is the prevention of dementia. Although there is no absolute way of preventing dementia, changes to lifestyle whilst younger or fitter can lower the risk of developing dementia when older. There are certain key areas that should be observed such as maintaining a healthy diet, in turn maintaining a healthy weight, which necessitates exercising regularly, being careful with alcohol consumption, quit (or don't start) smoking. Observing the above should help keep blood pressure at a level which lowers the risk of complications. In chapter 9 the importance of diet and exercise is discussed further.

Finding a cure for dementia

Researchers are hard at work trying to find the causes, and a subsequent cure for dementia. The causes of dementia have been outlined in the previous chapter. There are certain areas that scientists are concentrating on, outlined below:

Work around Gene Therapy

Gene therapy is an area of medicine in which genetic material is used to try to prevent or cure a particular disease. This is a relatively new area of research. In dementia, the aim of gene therapy is to stop brain cells dying, by replacing them if possible but this is still in its infancy and it may be a while before human trials begin.

Vaccines for dementia

This is also a relatively new area of research. A dementia vaccine would be a form of medication that would train the immune system to recognise the abnormal deposits of protein (such as amyloid plaques) in Alzheimer's disease that are thought to cause the damage to brain cells. The immune system would then attack these plaques, which might then slow the progress of the condition.

Stem cell treatment and dementia

Research into this kind of treatment is ongoing. Stem cells are known as 'building block' cells and they can develop into many different cell types, including brain cells. Currently, two main avenues of research into the use of stem cells are being explored. Firstly, stem cells are being manipulated so that they, in effect, mimic some of the body's processes that may cause the development of dementia. Secondly, researchers hope that stem cells, one day, can be used to develop new brain cells to replace the cells damaged by dementia. This type of research is also very beneficial to those with Parkinson's.

Dementia and psychology

As well as advances in medicine, there have also been important advances in the area of psychology. Cognitive stimulation is one area that is actively used and explored and involves people taking part in activities and exercises that are designed to improve memory, problem solving skills and also language ability. Validation therapy, as we have seen is an important area which is being advanced, where people are encouraged to explore what things were like for the person in the past and how this relates to the way they are feeling now.

There are also other areas in the field of psychology that are being explored, such as social media support groups. One of the aims of psychological intervention is to minimise the need for medications, in particular anti-psychotic medicines.

****

Chapter 3

The Day-to-Day Experience of Living and Coping With Dementia

Having looked at the nature of dementia and Alzheimer's, it is now necessary to address the many practical issues that arise once a person has been diagnosed with the condition. You may be the person suffering from dementia or the person caring for a dementia sufferer. Whatever the situation, there are certain very important issues that must be faced. The first of those are the practical considerations surrounding normal day-to-day living. In this chapter, we will also discuss holidays and breaks for people with dementia.

Day to day living-safety in the home

Not surprisingly, many people with dementia wish to stay in their own home for as long as possible, rather than go into a care home. In most cases, this will be with support from others. In Chapter Four we discuss the various types of home care available, including carers.

In this chapter, we concentrate on the practical aspects of ensuring a person with dementia is able to live and function securely in their own home and also, importantly be able to control their own legal and financial affairs.

Consulting an occupational therapist

One main aim is to make the home environment as safe as possible. In this respect, an occupational therapist can provide advice on the types of practical support a person might need to assist them to live comfortably. They can suggest ways to carry out daily living activities, i.e. bathing, eating and dressing safely. They can assist with participation in a wide range of activities to help with personal wellbeing, both psychological and spiritual. They can provide important advice to carers and also help with assistive technology.

What is assistive technology?

Assistive technology refers to devices or systems that support a person to maintain or improve their independence, safety and wellbeing. It tends to refer to devices and systems that assist people with memory problems or other cognitive difficulties, rather than those that are used to aid someone with mobility or physical difficulties.

Many assistive technology devices are electronic, but the term does not just refer to high-tech devices. However, devices such as smartphones and tablets, coupled with widespread internet coverage, are making technology more accessible for everyone in ways that we couldn't predict just a few years ago.

Widespread use of social media (such as Twitter and Facebook) also means that many people now live some of their life in a virtual environment, as well as in a more traditional face-to-face one.

Technology can be used in a variety of ways, and for a variety of purposes. It can support people in carrying out everyday tasks and activities, enhance a person's safety, support their social participation, and monitor their health. Assistive technology can help people who have problems with:

- speech
- hearing and eyesight
- safe walking
- finding their way around
- memory and cognition (thinking and understanding)
- daily living activities such as bathing and cooking meals
- socialising and leisure.

As mentioned, an occupational therapist can advise on the full range of assistive technologies that are available and that will be particularly suitable for a person with dementia. The Alzheimers Society will also offer invaluable advice and assitance in this area.

If you want to arrange an occupational therapy assessment you should speak to your GP or local social services department. If you would like a private occupational therapy assessment then you should contact the British Association of Occupational Therapists and College of Occupational Therapists www.cot.co.uk. Contact details along with other useful assistive technology organisations can be found in the useful resources section.

Avoidance of falls in the home

Falls are a problem which affects all older people. The risk will increase with the onset of dementia. There are a number of things that can be done at home to reduce the risk of falling:

- Home safety - Check the home for potential hazards such as rugs, loose carpets, furniture or objects lying on the floor.

- Exercise - Regular exercise can improve strength and balance and help to maintain good general health. A referral to a physiotherapist may also help.

- Healthy feet - Foot problems, including foot pain and long toenails, can contribute to an increased risk of falls. Seeing a podiatrist (a health professional who specialises in feet) can help. Contact your GP to find out more.

- Medicines - Medication can have side effects, including dizziness, which could increase the risk of a fall. Changes to medication or dosage, as well as taking multiple medicines, can increase a person's risk of falling. Speak to the GP about a medicine review if the person with dementia is taking more than four medicines.

- Eyesight - Regular eye tests and wearing the correct glasses may help to prevent falls.

- Keep objects in easy reach - If something is going to be used regularly, keep it in a cupboard or drawer that is easy to access.

- Try not to rush - Do things at an appropriate pace; many people fall when they are rushing.

Modifications to lighting in a home

Age related and visual impairment due to dementia can affect the way people can see and means that changes to lighting in a house will be necessary. Generally, as a person gets older their pupils get smaller, they have increased sensitivity to glare and there is a reduced amount of light reaching the retina. A person with dementia will have the added complication of damage to the visual system and this leads to difficulties. The actual difficulty will depend on the type of dementia, but may include:

- decreased sensitivity to differences in contrast (including colour contrast such as black and white, and contrast between objects and background)
- reduced ability to detect movement
- reduced ability to detect different colours (for example, a person may have problems telling the difference between blue and purple)
- changes to the visual field (how much someone can see around the edge of their vision while looking straight ahead)
- double vision.

Improved lighting can reduce falls, depression and sleep disorders, and improve independence and general health. The following tips may help:

- Increase light levels and use daylight where possible.
- Minimise glare, reflection and shadows. Glare can be distracting and can reduce a person's mobility.

- Lighting should be uniform across any space, and pools of light and sudden changes in light levels should be avoided. This is because when a person gets older, their eyes adapt slowly to changes in light levels.
- Remove visual clutter and distractions such as carpets with floral patterns.
- Use colour contrasts to make things clearer, for example a light door with a dark frame.
- Leave a light on in the toilet or bathroom during the night. A night light in the bedroom may help if someone gets up in the night.

Adaptations to the home

As people get older they may experience difficulties in managing everyday activities such as cooking or bathing, for a variety of reasons. People with dementia may experience additional challenges as their dementia progresses, because of memory problems or a reduced ability to carry out tasks in the correct sequence.

Adapting the Home can help people with dementia to maintain their independence and reduce the risk of harm. It can also help to adapt some everyday tasks slightly. The following tips may help:

- Label cupboards and objects with pictures and words so that they can be identified.
- Where possible, use devices that only have one function and are easy to identify, for example a kettle.

- Place clear instructions that can easily be followed somewhere visible.

- Make sure the kitchen is well-lit.

- If there are concerns about using gas or electrical appliances inappropriately, contact the gas or electricity company and ask for the person to be put on the priority service register. This means that they will be eligible for free regular safety checks and will be able to get advice about safety measures such as isolation valves (advice is also available for carers).

- Fit an isolation valve to a gas cooker so that the cooker cannot be turned on and left on. Devices are also available for electric cookers.

- Look into products that may help to maintain independence and safety such as electric kettles that switch off automatically.

- If the person's ability to recognise danger is declining, consider removing potentially dangerous implements such as sharp knives, but place other items for everyday use within easy reach.

Other tips for the maintenance of safety at home are:
- Store dangerous substances safely. This should always be the case anyway but especially so with dementia sufferers. If the person with dementia is unable to administer their own medication safely then arrangements should be made for someone else to do this. A dosette box would be helpful with separate tablet compartments for days of the

week, times of day etc. Your pharmacist should be able to advise on this.

- Avoid possible fires. Make sure smoke detetcors and carbon monoxide detectors are fitted. Also, check home appliances.

- Outdoor safety. Being outdoors is important for people of all ages and has many obvious benefits. Gardens or balconies can bring many benefits. However, it is important to manage any risks that may come with being outdoors. Make sure the area is well lit, this can be achieved with a sensor light. make sure that all stairs have a rail fitted, avoid trip hazards such as paving stones, have seating areas and make sure that there is adequate shelter, such as a gazebo or parasol over a table. These are all small things but will ensure that maximum safety can be achieved.

- Making sure that access is arranged. Ensure that someone has access in the event of a person with dementia or their carer being unable to answer the door. One option is a key safe fitted outside the home where keys are placed and which is coded. Social services can also advise on the provision of community alarms.

- Make sure that you have a complete record of phone numbers and names of everyone involved in the care of the person with dementia, such as the carer, GP, social worker etc.

- It may also help to list information such as:

- practical steps on who to contact and how to deal with an emergency, eg how to use an alert system

- any medications the person with dementia may need
- advice on strategies that work for the person with dementia if they become distressed, eg to aid communication or reduce anxiety
- where to find the gas and electricity meters, the fuse box and stopcock
- where to find the point to turn off the main gas supply
- location of the first aid box.

Tell anyone who might need this information where to find the list. You could also keep basic personal and medical details in an easy-to-access place in case of an emergency.

Incontinence

People with dementia commonly experience difficulties using the toilet, accidents on the way to the toilet and incontinence. Incontinence is the involuntary leakage of urine or faeces or both, which is known as double incontinence.

Urinary incontinence may be a small occasional leak or total loss of bladder control. The most common form in someone with dementia is an overactive bladder, where there is a suden intense need to go, and frequent urination. Women are at a particular risk of stress incontinence, when a cough, sneeze or laugh causes a small leak of urine.

Faecal incontinence may range from passing a small amount of stool when breaking wind, to having no bowel control at all. This is less common than urinary incontinence.

41

Incontinence is a common risk in older people in particular and is exacerbated by dementia. A carer can help by working with a person who has dementia by ensuring the following:

- The person should drink six to eight glasses of fluids each day - more if they have hard stools. Cutting down fluids or not drinking them for long periods of time (for example to avoid the need to urinate at night) can cause urinary tract infections and constipation.
- They should eat a balanced diet with at least five daily portions of fruit and vegetables, and enough fibre to ensure a regular bowel movement. See chapter 7.
- The person should keep as mobile as they can. If they are able, walking every day helps with bowel movements.
- Ensure a regular time, and allow enough time on the toilet, to empty bowels. There are biological reasons why trying to go a few minutes after a meal works - many people favour going after breakfast.

If a health professional has suggested the person might have an overactive bladder, they will also advise replacing drinks which irritate the bladder (eg tea, coffee, cola or alcohol) with water, herbal teas, squash and fruit drinks.

Women with mild dementia and urinary stress incontinence sometimes learn pelvic floor exercises, with the support of specialist continence nurses or physiotherapists. These exercises can cure stress incontinence caused by weakness of the pelvic floor muscles due to childbirth or ageing.

Constipation

If constipation is the problem, there are a wide range of laxitives available over the counter which will help relieve the problem. However, they should not be used for long periods without seeking advice from a GP. Carers can also massage a person's abdomen to help relieve the problem although this may not be to a person's liking.

The following ideas may help someone to find, recognise and use the toilet more easily:

- Help the person identify where the toilet is. A sign on the door, including both words and a picture, may help. Help the person know when the toilet is vacant; leaving the toilet door open when not in use makes this obvious.

- Help the person make their way easily to the toilet. Move any awkwardly placed furniture or prop ajar any doors that are hard to open. The room and the route to the toilet should be well lit, especially at night.

- Make using the toilet easier for people with mobility problems. Aids such as handrails and a raised toilet seat may help. Occupational therapists can give free advice on these, or you can ask someone at a local independent living shop.

- Help the person identify and use the toilet. A contrasting colour (eg black seat on a white base) can make it easier to see.

- Help the person undo, remove and replace clothing easily. Trousers with an elasticated waist (eg tracksuit bottoms) are often easier than zips. Some people find Velcro™ fastenings easier to use than zips or buttons.

- If getting to the toilet becomes too difficult because of mobility problems, an aid such as a commode may be useful. Using this will require the person to recognise the commode, be willing to use it, and find it an acceptable piece of furniture. PromoCon (see Useful resources at the back of the book) and independent living shops provide information on commodes and other aids. Alternatively, you can ask the occupational therapist, community nurse or social services.

- The person should have privacy in the toilet, but make sure they don't have difficulty managing locks. Some people with dementia struggle with this. To avoid the person locking themselves in, disable locks or ensure you can open them quickly from the outside.

Help when outside
There are several ways to make travelling or being outside easier for the person with dementia.

- Plan in advance. Find out where accessible toilets are.
- Go prepared. Fit a light pad (the kind that attaches to underwear) and carry spare clothing and pads, as well as a bag for soiled items.
- Buy a RADAR key (see useful Resources). This gives disabled people - including people with dementia - independent access to thousands of locked public toilets around the country.

- Carry a Just Can't Wait toilet card. These can be bought from the Bladder and Bowel Foundation (see Useful Resources). The card should encourage places such as shops to help with access to toilets. Use the disabled toilet if the person needs you to help them with the toilet (particularly if you are of a different gender).

Help with scheduled use of the toilet

For someone who is regularly wet it may be better to develop a timetable to offer help or reminders for going to the toilet, for example when they wake up, before each meal, at morning and afternoon coffee or tea, and before bed. For faecal incontinence, it is often possible to re-establish continence by going to the toilet at a set time each day and helping the person stay long enough to have a bowel movement.

Professional support

The GP should be the first port of call. The doctor should review the symptoms and any underlying medical conditions (eg urinary tract infection or constipation), diet or medications that might be causing the problems. The doctor may do an internal examination of the bowel.

If this assessment is unable to resolve things, ask to have the person referred to a continence adviser. You may have to be persistent here: NHS continence services across the country are quite variable and you may have to push to see someone who understands incontinence in people with dementia. There may be a wait for these services. After a thorough assessment the continence adviser will write up a continence care plan tailored to the individual. The plan should include things that the person with dementia and any carer can do to help. It should also describe the support that professionals should provide, as well as follow-up and next steps.

In a few cases referral to further specialists (eg geriatrician, urologist or gynaecologist) will be needed. For some people, advice will focus not on cure but on containing the incontinence as comfortably as possible using aids. Other health professionals can visit at home and offer support:

- A community nurse can help with access to NHS-funded continence products and advise on management, hygiene and how to protect the skin.
- An occupational therapist can advise on adaptations and equipment.
- A physiotherapist can advise if manual dexterity is the problem.
- A community psychiatric nurse, Admiral Nurse or the community mental health team can help if behavioural changes are affecting how someone uses the toilet.

Ask the GP about being referred to these professionals.

Driving and dementia

Someone who is diagnosed with dementia may be able to continue driving for some time. However, they must fulfil certain legal requirements. As the person's dementia progresses, they will reach a point where they can no longer drive safely and must stop driving. The DVLA and also the Alzheimers Society offer advice on the position of a person with dementia and the continued ability to drive.

A person must fulfil certain legal requirements, including telling the Driver and Vehicle Licensing Agency (DVLA) in England, Scotland and Wales, or Driver and Vehicle Licensing Northern Ireland (DVLNI) in Northern Ireland, of their diagnosis.

To drive, a person needs to be able to:
- make sense of and respond to everything they see - including road signs and obstacles
- maintain attention while 'reading the road'
- anticipate and react quickly to the actions of other road users
- take appropriate action (eg braking, steering) to avoid accidents
- plan and remember where they are going.

Many people with dementia retain learned skills and are able to drive safely for some time after diagnosis. However, as dementia progresses beyond the early stages it has serious effects on memory, reactions, perception and the ability to perform even simple tasks. People with dementia will, therefore, eventually lose the ability to drive. The stage at which this happens will be different for each person but, according to research, most people stop driving within three years after the first signs of the disease.

People taking certain types of medication, such as night sedation or drugs for depression, may also find that their driving ability is affected. Advice should be obtained from a GP if this is the case.

If, following its enquiries, DVLA/DVLNI decides that the person cannot continue driving, the person must return their driving licence to DVLA/DVLNI and stop driving. However, there is an appeal process. A formal appeal must be lodged with the Magistrates' Court within six months in England and Wales. In Northern Ireland an appeal must be lodged with the appropriate Clerk of Petty Sessions within three months. Someone who has appealed against removal of their licence is not allowed to drive in the meantime.

Below are the addresses of the DVLA offices in the UK:

Driver and Vehicle Licensing Agency (DVLA)
Swansea SA99 1TU
T 0300 790 6806 (Monday to Friday 8.00am-5.30pm, Saturday 8.00am-1.00pm)
E eftd@dvla.gsi.gov.uk
W www.dft.gov.uk/dvla/medical
www.gov.uk/dementia-and-driving (Questionnaire form for those with a medical condition that will affect their driving)

Driver and Vehicle Licensing Agency (DVLA)
CCG Drivers
Swansea SA6 7JL
T 0300 790 6801
W www.dft.gov.uk/dvla
www.gov.uk/contact-the-dvla

Driver and Vehicle Licensing Northern Ireland (DVLNI)
Castlerock Road
Coleraine BT51 3TB
T 0845 4024 000
E dvlni@doeni.gov.uk
W www.dvlni.gov.uk

In addition, the Alzheimer's Society and Citizens Advice Bureau can offer further advice.

Employment and dementia

If you are working, you may be having problems at work as a result of your dementia. When you feel ready, speak to your employer about your diagnosis. It will be easier if they are involved from the beginning.

You can get advice and support from your trade union, your local Citizens Advice Bureau or from the disability employment adviser at your local job centre. You can also discuss the effect that dementia has on your work with your GP or consultant. If you decide to carry on working, your employer should consider what they can do to help. They might, for example, consider reducing your hours or changing your job.

However, you may decide to leave work. If this is the case, it is important not to feel as though you are giving up. Before you leave employment, seek advice on your pension and social security benefits rights.

Holidays for people with dementia

Going on holiday should be a relaxing and enjoyable experience. This is no different for people with dementia and their friends and family. There are lots of benefits to a holiday, such as having new experiences and giving the person with dementia and those close to them a break from routine. However, dementia can make it more difficult to travel.

The Alzheimer's Society factsheets give very useful tips and advice about planning a holiday for people affected by dementia, including choosing the right type of holiday and arranging travel insurance and medical care. It also explains the best ways to get around and any financial help that is available for taking a holiday. The topics covered in the factsheets include:

- Planning a holiday
- What type of holiday to take, for example staying with friends or relatives or specialist travel. There are companies that exist to provide holidays for people with dementia, see useful resources at the back of the book.
- Planning your holiday: tips for carers
- Knowing your rights
- Preparing and packing
- Passport and other identification documents
- Medicines
- Travel insurance
- The European Health Insurance Card
- Treatment in countries outside the EEA

- The journey
- Travelling by air
- Travelling by coach or bus
- Travelling by sea
- Travelling by car
- Arrival: Tips for carers
- Financial assistance

There is a wide range of information which can help you decide whether you want to go on holiday and whether it would be beneficial to you or, if you are a carer, to the person with dementia.

End of life care

People with dementia often live for many years after their diagnosis. The symptoms of dementia are likely to get worse over time, and it's wise to make plans well in advance of a person's condition deteriorating.

People with an incurable illness such as dementia, may be offered so-called end of life care (or palliative care) so they are able to live as well as possible until their death. End of life care also includes support for family members. Care can be provided at home, in a hospice, a care home, or hospital.

Everyone who has been diagnosed with dementia should have a care plan drawn up with healthcare professionals. End of life care should be a key part of this dementia care plan. Details of end of life care included in the dementia care plan might include the person with dementia specifying where they would like to die, and how they'd like to be treated. The dementia care plan should also provide some support for carers, who will be grieving around the time of death.

Preferences for end of life care should ideally be discussed and set out soon after a diagnosis of dementia. Actions such as making an advance statement of wishes should be thought about as soon as possible.

Care at home for people with advanced dementia

Palliative care services may sometimes be offered in the home, rather than in a hospice building. "Hospice-at-home" services have staff that are usually on call 24 hours a day and can visit people at home. Your GP can arrange for community palliative care nurses to provide care in the home. Your local authority may also provide social care services and equipment for the home.

Hospices are specialist residential units run by a team of doctors, nurses, social workers, counsellors and trained volunteers. They are smaller and quieter than hospitals and feel more like a home. Hospices can provide individual care more suited to individuals in a gentler, calmer atmosphere. There is no charge for hospice care, but patients must be referred to a hospice through their GP.

Palliative care in a care home

Palliative care is available in residential care homes. If someone with dementia is already in a residential home, they may want to stay there for their palliative care. This may make them more comfortable and less distressed than having to go into hospital, unless that is necessary.

You should ask if the residential home is accredited by the end of life Gold Standards network, which means that the home has specially trained staff and good links with local GPs.

Palliative care for dementia as a hospice day patient

If someone who has dementia prefers to remain living at home, they may be able to visit a hospice during the day. This means they can receive the care and support they need without permanently leaving their home.

As a day patient, they will be able to access more services than could be offered if they stayed at home. Such services might include creative and complementary therapies and rehabilitation, as well as nursing and medical care. They will also meet other patients. Hospices often provide transport to and from the hospice.

See useful resources for organisations dealing with End-of-Life Care.

The importance of exercise and diet

Exercise and diet play an important part in anyone's life. They play a particularly important part in the life of someone with dementia. It is recognised that it is difficult for someone with dementia to exercise adequately. Nevertheless there are exercises that can be carried out effectively that will help and assist a person to stay mentally and physically healthier. In Chapter 8 we discuss diet and exercise in depth.

In the next chapter, we will look at aspects of financial and legal management and how they affect a person with dementia.

****

Chapter 4

Financial and Legal Management

In the previous chapter, we looked at the practical aspects of managing day-to-day activities, and the overall home environment. Before we look at accessing support and the wide range of services available to dementia sufferers and their families, another area of immediate concern that needs to be addressed is the management of finances and financial affairs, plus the management of legal affairs, which impacts on medical care. As a person becomes less able to look after their own affairs, this leaves them vulnerable to exploitation or to the consequences of mis-management.

Planning for the future

There may come a time when a person with dementia is no longer able to make certain decisions for themselves. In England and Wales a law called the Mental Capacity Act 2005 sets out what should happen when someone is able to make these decisions for themselves (known as having 'mental capacity') and when they are not. The Citizens Advice website provides details of respective laws dealing with mental capacity in Scotland and Northern Ireland.

The Act also provides ways for someone to plan ahead for their future, should there come a time when they lose mental capacity.

There are a number of ways to plan ahead for this eventuality; collectively these are referred to as 'advance care planning'. They include making decisions about future care and treatment, who could make decisions on their behalf, or who might manage their finances if they were unable to do this for themselves. You can get more advice about the Mental Capacity Act, and what it means, from a Citizens Advice Bureau or from the Alzheimers Society. Below we will look at becoming a deputy for a person and also obtaining Lasting Power of Attorney, which are key ways of ensuring a person is protected.

Becoming a deputy for someone with Dementia

If a person with dementia has not already got in place a plan for their own future decision making, and the carer, whoever that may be (not a paid carer, due to conflicts of interest), feels that they need to make decisions on their behalf, then they can apply to the Court of Protection to become their deputy. Becoming a deputy involves a lot of ongoing responsibility, and these responsibilities continue into the future.

A deputy is usually a friend or relative of the person who lacks capacity. However, in certain circumstances it could be a professional such as a solicitor or accountant or another person appointed by the court. Professional deputies charge fees for their time which is paid by the person with dementia or out of their estate. To become a deputy you need to be at least 18 years of age and willing to be a deputy. There are two different types of deputyship-property and affairs and personal welfare.

Property and affairs deputyship

A property and affairs deputyship is the most common type of deputyship. Someone will apply to become a deputy if they feel that there is a need to manage the financial affairs of the person with dementia and there is not a Lasting Power of Attorney in place (see below). Also, there must be something to manage, for example if the person is in receipt of benefits and this is the only source of income then a deputy will not usually be needed. The benefits can be managed by an appointee from the Department of Works and Pensions, www.gov.uk/dwp.

When applying to become a deputy the court will want to see that you are a fit and able person and that you have the skills and knowledge to manage the person's affairs and, for example, you do not have any financial problems yourself which might compromise your trustworthiness.

Personal welfare deputyship

This type of deputyship is rare. If a person lacks the capacity to make decisions about their own care and treatment and has not appointed an attorney, someone must apply to become a deputy if they feel the need to manage that person's personal affairs. The Court of Protection does not usually appoint deputies to make continuing decisions about someone's health and welfare unless regular treatment and supervision is needed. These decisions can usually be made on the person's behalf by whoever is providing the treatment. If there is a disagreement about the treatment then it may be necessary to ask the court to intervene although this is rare given the levels of consultation between health professionals and dementia patients and their carers.

Legal matters-Lasting Powers of Attorney

Many people with dementia will eventually reach a point where they are no longer able to make decisions for themselves – this is known as lacking 'mental capacity'. When this happens, someone else – often a carer or family member – will need to make decisions on their behalf. A Lasting Power of Attorney (LPA) is a legal tool that gives another adult the legal authority to make certain decisions for you, if you become unable to make them yourself. The person who is given this authority is known as an 'attorney'. They can manage your finances, or make decisions relating to your health and welfare.

As with Deputyships, there are two different types of LPA. One of them covers decisions about your property and finances, and the other covers decisions about your health and welfare. You can choose to make both types or just one. You can appoint the same person to be your attorney for both, or you can have different attorneys. An LPA can only be used after it has been registered at the Office of the Public Guardian (OPG). The OPG is responsible for the registration of LPAs

Benefits of making an LPA

It can be reassuring to know that, if you are unable to make a decision for yourself in the future, the person you choose will make these decisions for you. Making an LPA ensures that the person you want to make decisions for you will be able to do so.

This prevents a stranger, or someone you may not trust, from having this power.

Who can make an LPA?

Anyone who is over the age of 18 and has the mental capacity to do so can make an LPA. Once a person has lost mental capacity, they will not be able to appoint an LPA. If the person's family or friends then want to be able to make certain decisions on their behalf, they will need to apply for deputyship.

Who can be an attorney?

You can choose anyone you want to be your attorney, as long as they are over 18. For a property and affairs LPA, however, the person you choose cannot be bankrupt. It's important to think carefully about who to appoint. Think about who knows you well and who you trust to make these decisions for you, and also whether the person is reliable and has the skills to carry out the role. You can choose to have more than one attorney.

Most people will choose a relative or close friend to be their attorney, especially for a health and welfare LPA. You can also ask a professional however, such as an accountant or solicitor. You might want to think about whether this would be a good option for a property and affairs LPA. A professional may charge for their time, and you need to name an individual rather than an organisation or company. The person must also be willing and able to carry out the role. You can also appoint a replacement attorney. This is the person who you would want to make decisions for you if your first choice of attorney is no longer able or willing to carry out their role. You might want to think about this, especially if you are only appointing one person to act as your attorney.

It is worth noting here that the legal profession makes a lot of money charging high fees for dealing with the setting up of LPA's. There are advice services you can access to minimise costs. There is one service, set up by a man whose mother suffered from Dementia, called Unforgettable www.unforgettable.org which helps those in a similar position through the maze of applying for an LPA.

For more information concerning how to apply to become a deputy and also Lasting Powers of Attorney you should contact the below:

Court of Protection
PO Box 70185
First Avenue House
42-49 High Holborn
London WC1A 9JA
T 0300 456 4600
E courtofprotectionenquiries@hmcts.gsi.gov.uk
W www.gov.uk/apply-to-the-court-of-protection

The Court of Protection makes decisions and appoints deputies to act on behalf of people who are unable to make decisions about their personal health, finance or welfare.

Office of the Public Guardian
PO Box 16185
Birmingham B2 2WH
T 0300 456 0300 (customer services, 9am-5pm weekdays)
E customerservices@publicguardian.gsi.gov.uk
W www.gov.uk/browse/births-deaths-marriages/lasting-power-attorney

The OPG supervises deputies, and are able to provide deputies with guidance and support.

Solicitors for the Elderly
Solicitors for the Elderly Ltd
Room 17, Conbar House
Mead Lane
Hertford SG13 7AP
T 0844 5676 173
E admin@solicitorsfortheelderly.com

Solicitors for the Elderly is an independent, national organisation of lawyers, such as solicitors, barristers, and legal executives who provide specialist legal advice for older and vulnerable people, their families and carers.

In addition, the Alzheimers Society and Age UK provide detailed information concerning the role of deputies and Lasting Powers of Attorney and how to apply together with ongoing responsibilities.

Northern Ireland

To give someone power of attorney in Northern Ireland you will need to make an Eduring Power of Attorney. Again, the Alzheimer's Society or the Citizens Advice Bureaucan can provide more information.

Other financial matters

There are other financial matters that need to be taken care of when helping a person with dementia. Welfare benefits are covered in-depth in Chapter 7. In addition, both Age UK and the Alzheimer's Society plus the Citizens Advice Bureau provide advice on the various benefits available. Other areas to be taken care of are bank accounts and items such as direct debits and standing orders, Joint accounts, wills and trusts plus access to bank accounts.

Third-party mandate

A third-party mandate enables an account holder to nominate someone to have access to their bank account. This can allow a person with dementia to get support with their account, or let the nominated person pay bills or visit the bank on their behalf. It's important that the account holder nominates someone they trust.

The bank can advise on setting up a third-party mandate.

Chip and signature bank cards

For someone concerned about remembering their personal identification number (PIN) for their bank card, a chip and signature card may be helpful. This works like a normal bank card, but instead of having to put a PIN into a machine, the holder is asked to sign a receipt, and their signature is checked.

The bank can give information on getting a chip and signature card. They can also advise on any implications this might have. For example, not all chip and signature cards enable someone to access money from a cash machine, so the person will have to go into the bank for cash. Also, chip and signature cards are generally not accepted at self-service checkouts.

Joint-accounts

Some people find that joint bank accounts can be helpful in the short term. They allow both the person and another account holder to access and manage the account. Often people have a joint bank account with their partner or a child. A joint bank account can give a person with dementia peace of mind that someone else is supporting them with organising bills and payments. Your bank will assist you or the person you are caring for in setting up a joint account. They will also let you know the advantages and disadvantages of holding a joint account.

Wills

It is always advisable to make a will; it ensures that when someone dies, their money and possessions go to people they have chosen. Someone who has received a diagnosis of dementia may wish to make or change a will. They should seek legal advice from a solicitor as soon as possible. A diagnosis of dementia doesn't necessarily mean that someone can't make a will. It depends whether they have 'testamentary capacity'. This is the legal capacity to make or change their will. The solicitor will make a decision about this, often after taking medical advice.

Trusts

Some people consider setting up a trust if they have financial assets such as property or savings. This ensures that the assets are managed in a way that the person chooses, now and in the future. There are a number of different kinds of trusts and ways of arranging them.

This can be complex; consulting a solicitor or qualified financial adviser may help. It is important that the trust is set up well ahead of a time when the person may need care in a care home. This is because the local authority needs to be sure that they have not set up a trust to deliberately avoid contributing towards the cost of their care.

****

Chapter 5

Wider Help and Support-Social Services, NHS, Carers and Support Networks Generally

---

One of the most important areas to understand when you, or someone you care for, has been diagnosed with a form of dementia, is the wide range of help available to you, for example from the local authority, social services and the NHS. You will want to know:

- how a person can get specialist help in their home, what role social services play in providing this help,
- How to designate a carer and what support he or she can receive,
- how is the help funded, i.e. does the local authority pay, does the NHS pay, or do you pay yourself?
- If you are a young person with dementia, what services are available to you?

In the next two chapters, we will cover all aspects of care, beginning with the role of the NHS.

NHS care
Most people will already have used the health service in their area, in one way or another. You might also have attended a memory clinic. The aims of the Memory Clinic are: to give an in-

depth assessment of the person's memory function and cognition (thinking processes) to make a diagnosis. Your local NHS dementia service can supply more details about memory clinics. There are a wide range of other professionals within the NHS who can help such as:

- A range of mecdical specialists, for example psychiatrists, geriaticians and neurologists
- Nurses and community nurses
- Psychologists who can assess memory problems and also advise on talking therapies
- Audiologists for hearing problems
- Optomotrists for sight problems
- Dentists
- Physiotherapists
- Chiropodists
- Occupational therapists
- Speech and language therapists
- Counsellors
- Dietitians

As you can see, there is a wide variety of expertise within the NHS which will be of invaluable help and support to a person with dementia.

Although many services are centered around older people, the NHS will also provide help and support to young people with dementia. To obtain information about these services you should contact your GP or social services.

Carers and Dementia

What is a Carer?

A carer is anyone who cares, unpaid, for a friend or family member who due to illness, disability, a mental health problem or an addiction cannot cope without their support. The causes of someone taking on caring responsibilities include:

o   Serious physical illness
o   Long-term physical disability
o   Long-term neurological conditions
o   Mental health problems
o   Dementia
o   Addiction
o   Learning difficulties

This support could include being offered money to pay for things that make caring easier. Or the local authority might offer practical support, such as arranging for someone to step in when you need a short break. It could also put you in touch with local support groups so you have people to talk to.

The Care Act 2014

The Care Act 2014, which was given Royal assent in May 2014, makes carer's assessments more widely available to people in caring roles. Local authorities now have a legal duty to assess any carer who requests one or who appears to need support. If you are a carer and you need some support, you should get in touch with the council covering the area where the person you care for lives. The council will provide you with information and advice about how the assessment will work.

Essentially, a Carer's assessment is a discussion between you and a trained person either from the council or another organisation that the council works with. The assessment will consider the impact the care and support you provide is having on your own wellbeing, as well as important aspects of the rest of your life, including the things you want to achieve day-to-day. It must also consider other important issues, such as whether you are able or willing to carry on caring, whether you work or want to work, and whether you want to study or do more socially. The assessment can be carried out face-to-face, over the telephone or online.

When the assessment is complete, the local authority will decide whether your needs are "eligible" for support from the local authority. After the assessment, they will write to you about their decision and give you reasons to explain what they have decided. If you have eligible needs, your council will contact you to discuss what help might be available. If you do not have needs that are eligible, your council will give you information and advice, including what local care and support is available. This could include, for example, help from local voluntary organisations.

As well as care and support organised by the council, some people are also eligible to receive help from the NHS. This help may be a nursing service for people who are ill or recovering at home after leaving hospital. It could include things like changing the dressings on wounds or giving medication. If you are eligible for this kind of help, a health professional such as your GP or community nurse should be able to tell you.

In exceptional circumstances, where an adult has a complex medical condition and substantial ongoing care needs, the NHS provides a service called NHS continuing healthcare. NHS continuing healthcare provides care and support in a person's home, care home or hospice.

In order to get more details concerning a carers role and rights and responsibilities you should contact your local authority. In addition, organisations such as Carers UK (see useful resources) can assist you.

What social care services are available?
Having identified the role of a carer, and how to get help, it is important to understand the wide variety of services available to dementia sufferers. Before we look at receiving an assessment from social services we will detail the different types of care available.

There are a wide variety of social care services available to dementia sufferers and most people will be able to have care provided in their home. The kind of social care support you can get depends largely on your needs. This means the type of condition you have, or the severity of your disability. These needs will usually be assessed through a *care assessment*, discussed in Chapter 6.

Care and support services available might typically include provison of equipment, help in your home, community support and activities and a range of other help from home adaptations to financial support. Your local authority will be able to provide more information concerning the range of services available.

Obtaining help in your home

You may want to have someone who can come to your home and give you the support you need to live your life. This can include help with tasks such as getting dressed, help with using the toilet, washing, preparing and eating food, cleaning and laundry, getting out and about, and taking part in leisure and social activities.

Types of homecare

Homecare comes in a number of forms including home help, care attendants and "carers". Homecare can suit you if you need personal care, such as washing or dressing, housekeeping or domestic work, such as vacuuming, cooking or preparing meals, nursing and health care and companionship.

Homecare can be very flexible, in order to meet required needs, and the same person or agency may be able to provide some or all of the below options for the duration of your care:

- long-term 24-hour care
- short breaks for an unpaid family carer
- emergency care
- day care
- sessions ranging from 15-minute visits to 24-hour assistance and everything in between

A good source of information is the NHS Choices directories www.nhs.co.uk which lists homecare services and agencies local to you as well as national organisations which will advise on financial and practical support and can also advise on "shared lives" services where you can find a place to live with a family. In addition, if you are eligible for homecare services, the local authority may provide or arrange the help themselves. Alternatively, you can arrange your own care, funded by the local authority, through direct payments or a personal budget (see Chapter 6).

Independent homecare agencies

If you use an independent homecare agency, you or the person you're looking after has to find the care agency and pay them. The agency will provide a service through a trained team of care workers, which means you may not always have the same person visiting your home, although the agency will do its best to take your choices into account. Independent homecare providers are regulated by the Care Quality Commission (CQC) www.cqc.org.uk. Homecare agencies must meet CQC's national minimum standards and regulations in areas such as training and record-keeping. The CQC has the power to inspect agencies and enforce standards.

An agency will want to see you and the person you're looking after so that they can assess your needs. This also means that a joint decision can be made about the most appropriate type of care and support. You can find out more about agencies from the UK Homecare Association www.ukhca.co.uk.

Disadvantages of using a homecare agency

The main disadvantage is the cost of using an agency. The agency will charge a fee on top of the payment made to the care worker to cover their running costs and profit. You normally have to make a regular payment to the agency, which includes both the worker's earnings and the agency's fee.

Homecare from charities

Charities such as Age UK and Carers Trust (addresses and websites at back of the book in the Useful Resources section), can provide home help and domestic assistance services. The Carers Trust supports carers by giving them a break from their caring responsibilities.

Community support and activities available to you

Some social care services can be provided to help you, or the person you are caring for, continue to play an active role in the community and to get out and about and do the things you want to do.

For example, you may want to work or to partake in religious or cultural events. Social care services may be able to support you in a wide range of ways to enable you to continue to do these things, for example a community transport service. Day centres provide meals and an opportunity to socialise and do activities that might not be available at home and may provide respite for family carers. You should also think about the possibility of taking holidays which can be very therapeutic for a dementia sufferer and families/carers.

Adaptations to your home

A common way that social care can support ill or disabled people to live independently at home is simple adaptations to the home. If you, or the person you are caring for, has difficulty living at home because of their/your condition, it is often a better option to improve ther home than to move somewhere new. For example, depending on the condition, you might be able to get lowered kitchen surfaces and storage, wider doorways to accommodate wheelchairs or walking frames, or improved flooring to prevent trips and falls.

Residential care

If living at home is no longer a realistic or practical option, you may want to consider residential care. There are many different types of 'residential care' – it may mean a permanent move into a care home for older people, or it could be a stay in a home for younger adults. Residential care may be privately owned, or run by a charity or the local authority. The main types of residential options are:

- residential care homes
- residential care homes with nursing care
- extra care and sheltered housing
- supported living
- retirement villages

Deciding on a long-term stay in residential care is a significant decision financially, practically and emotionally. You will need to think about your own preferences, or the preferences of the person you are caring for, and decide what services will meet your needs, as well as being flexible enough to take account of future care needs. In addition to your local authority, many local and national charities will also be able to provide information and advice.

Information and advisory services

People who need care may have difficulty in being able to exert their rights, get the services they need and are entitled to, or simply not know or understand what is available to them. Information and advice are often a key part of any care assessment that your local authority undertakes. This information could go a long way to helping you get the support you need. Charities are a major source of social care information – particularly those associated with conditions, such as the Alzheimer's Society, Mind, or Scope and also those related to different aspects of care, such as Carers UK or Independent Age (addresses and websites in the Useful Resources section). There are also Advocacy Services.

Advocacy services

Advocacy services help people – particularly those who are most vulnerable in society – to:

- access information and services
- be involved in decisions about their lives
- explore choices and options
- defend and promote their rights and responsibilities
- speak out about issues that matter to them

An advocacy service is provided by an advocate who is independent of social services and the NHS, and who isn't part of your family or one of your friends. An advocate's role includes arguing your case when you need them to, and making sure the correct procedures are followed by your health and social care services. Local authorities fund advocacy services in their area. To find an advocacy service, contact your local council or check its website. If you have a care co-ordinator from your local social services or healthcare team, they will liaise with other agencies for you.

Advocacy and mental capacity

The Mental Capacity Act 2005 introduced Independent Mental Capacity Advocates (IMCAs). An IMCA supports people who can't make or understand decisions by stating their views and wishes or securing their rights. This is a statutory advocacy service, which means in certain situations people who lack capacity must be referred to an advocate.An IMCA is not the decision-maker (such as the person's doctor or care manager), but the decision-maker has a duty to take into account the information given by the IMCA.

The Independent Mental Capacity Advocate (IMCA) service aims to help particularly vulnerable people who otherwise have no family or friends consult about those decisions. GOV.UK has more information on what it means to have an IMCA.

Independent advocates under the Care Act
The IMCA service is not the only form of independent advocacy available to support individuals. New advocacy provision has been introduced as part of the Care Act 2014.

The Care Act introduced new statutory advocacy from April 2015. This is for people who have substantial difficulty in being involved with the assessment of their needs, or with their care planning or care reviews, if they have nobody appropriate to help them be engaged. Your local authority can provide more information.

Having identified areas where you could possibly get help the next step is to arrange an assessment of your needs, which will result in a care and support plan.

****

Chapter 6

Care and Support Plans for Dementia Sufferers

In the previous chapter, we looked at the wide range of services available to a person with dementia. If you need non-medical support at home, the first step is to ask social services for a needs assessment, also called a community care assessment. This will provide a structured plan and also allow you to access vital services and in many cases to receive funding.

In order to receive an assessment of your needs, or the needs of the person suffering with Dementia you will need, or someone on your behalf will need, to contact your local social services. If you are assessed by social services and are found to be eligible for support, the next stage is to draw up a care and support plan. A care plan sets out how your care and support needs will be met. You should be fully involved in the preparation of your care plan, and you and anyone else you request should also get a written copy. The care plan must set out:

- the needs identified by the assessment
- whether, and to what extent, the needs meet the eligibility criteria
- the needs that the authority is going to meet, and how it intends to do so
- for a person needing care, for which of the desired outcomes care and support could be relevant

- for a carer, the outcomes the carer wishes to achieve, and their wishes around providing care, work, education and recreation where support could be relevant
- the personal budget
- information and advice on what can be done to reduce the needs in question, and to prevent or delay the development of needs in the future
- where needs are being met via a direct payment, the needs to be met via the direct payment and the amount and frequency of the payments

Your care plan should be individual to you, and you should be allowed to have as much involvement in the development of your plan as you wish. Care and support should help you to live independently, have as much control over your life as possible, participate in society on an equal level, with access to employment and a family life, have the best possible quality of life and keep as much dignity and respect as possible.

Reviews of your care plan

Your care plan should be reviewed by social services within the first three months, and then at least annually. The review looks at whether the outcomes identified in the care plan are being met. It should also review these goals to make sure they're still appropriate and check that any risk assessments are up to date.

Challenging your care plan

If you're not happy with a care plan, the services provided, or the way an assessment was carried out, you will need to use the local authority's complaints process. It can sometimes be helpful to get support when you're making a complaint. Sources of help can include an advocacy organisation which we discussed in the previous chapter.

Funding care-local authority funding for care

There are some services the local authority provides that it cannot charge for. But for many services, the local authority may carry out a financial assessment to see if you should pay for, or contribute to, the cost of your care services. Local authorities are not required to charge for care services, but they must abide by legal guidance if they do.

Services local authorities must provide free of charge

There are some items the local authority must provide for free if you are assessed as needing them. These are community equipment, minor adaptations to your home and reablement.

Community equipment

"Community equipment" means items specifically designed to make daily life easier for you. For example equipment to help with zips or buttons, telephones with large buttons or flashing lights communication aids and telecare equipment. A local authority may have set rules about the type of equipment it will consider supplying, or the level of costs it will meet.

Minor adaptations

Minor adaptations costing less than £1,000 are provided by local authorities at no charge. Minor adaptations include grab rails to make it safer to get in and out of a bath, blocks to make beds higher, raised toilet seats and bath seats. In some cases you may be asked to pay associated costs, such as maintenance charges. If you disagree with the decision about a minor adaptation, use the complaints procedure. If the adaptation will cost more than £1,000, you may be eligible for a disabled facilities grant.

Reablement

Reablement services are meant to help people adapt to a recent illness or disability by learning or relearning the skills necessary for independent daily living at home. Reablement services may be offered to someone who has recently come out of hospital. It can include helping you practise daily activities such as cooking and bathing to help you regain skills and get your confidence back.

Reablement should be provided free of charge by the local authority for up to six weeks. In some cases the support may be expected to last longer than six weeks – for instance, if someone has recently become sight impaired – and the local authority should consider the benefits of this, including the reduced risk of hospital readmissions.

Financial assessment for care and support services

If you have been assessed as needing care services, your local authority will carry out a financial assessment (a means test) to see if you should pay something towards the cost of your care. This assessment looks at your income, including tax credits and some benefits after disability-related expenses (if it is including disability benefits). Disability-related expenditure can include items such as laundry, maintenance, respite care, and extra bedding.

If you need to go into a care home, the local authority must ensure you have enough money to spend on any personal items you might need, such as clothes and toiletries. This is known as a personal expenses allowance (PEA).

A local authority has the discretion to allow a larger personal expenses allowance – for example, if you have dependent children, or you are a temporary resident and also need to meet the costs of your own property. If you'd experience hardship if the allowance was not increased, you should complain about this to the local authority.

If you are receiving care in your own home, the local authority must ensure you have enough money left after charges to meet your living costs, such as rent and food. This is known as the minimum income guarantee (MIG). The levels are the equivalent of Income Support plus 25%, and the amounts are set out in regulations.

Capital rules

The local authority will also look at your capital, such as savings and property. Currently, local authorities won't contribute to the cost of your care if you have more than £23,250 in savings and property (known as "capital"). From April 2020, this threshold will rise alongside the introduction of the cap on care costs, so more people will be eligible for help sooner. Support is means-tested, which means the local authority will carry out a financial assessment to work out what you can afford to contribute towards the cost of your care. If you have more than this capital limit because of the value of your home, but you have a low income, the local authority may allow you to defer payment while you arrange to sell your home.

If you are receiving local authority support with the cost of your care and you need to live in a certain place to receive that care, such as a care home, you have the right to choose where you live (choice of accommodation). The local authority must ensure you have at least one choice that is affordable from the amount identified in your personal budget, and ideally more than one. Some local authorities will have a list of preferred providers that they will usually recommend.

You may choose a care home that is more expensive than the amount set out in your personal budget. If you do, a third party such as a relative or friend must be willing and able to pay the difference in cost for the likely duration of your stay. This is known as a top-up payment.

Where a person agrees to enter into a top-up payment, they will need to sign a written agreement with the local authority. This will set out what the costs are, how often they have to be paid, and what will happen if the person is no longer able to make the payment. In some limited circumstances you can make this payment. This is if you enter into a deferred payment scheme, or you benefit from the value of your property being disregarded for the first 12 weeks of your care. The restrictions on paying this additional cost yourself will be lifted from April 2020, when the point at which means-tested support for care costs is increased.

The local authority can never require you to pay a top-up payment and must ensure there is at least one choice available within the amount set in your personal budget. Any arrangements to pay a top-up must involve your local authority, and should not be directly between you and your provider.

Alternative funding

There are alternatives to care funded by the local authority, for example NHS care. The NHS is responsible for funding certain types of healthcare equipment you may need. In some situations, the NHS is also responsible for meeting care needs. This is usually when your need is mainly for healthcare rather than social care. NHS care could be provided in hospital, but it could be in someone's own home or elsewhere in the community.

NHS continuing healthcare

If the person you care for has very severe and complex health needs, they may qualify for NHS Continuing Healthcare. This is an ongoing package of care that's fully funded by the NHS. In some areas of the country, you can arrange your NHS Continuing Healthcare using a personal health budget – similar to the personal budgets for social care outlined above.

NHS-funded nursing care

You should receive NHS-funded nursing care if:

- you live in a care home registered to provide nursing care, and

- you don't qualify for NHS Continuing Healthcare but have been assessed as needing care from a registered nurse

The NHS will make a payment directly to the care home to fund care from registered nurses who are usually employed by the care home.

NHS aftercare

People who were previously detained in hospital under certain sections of the Mental Health Act will have their aftercare services provided for free.

Help from charities and funds

There are other sources of funding you might be able to access to help you with funding care. Some charities can help with funding care needs. The cost of care and support is likely to be a long-term commitment and may be substantial, particularly if you choose to go into a care home, or if you have care needs at an early age. If you or a member of the family need to pay for care at home or in a care home, it's important to understand the alternatives. This makes advice tailored to your individual needs vital. You can get advice from:

- your local authority – through an assessment of your care and support needs, as well as advice on which services are available locally

- financial advice from a qualified, independent source – there are independent financial advisers who specialise in care funding advice; they are regulated by the Financial Conduct Authority and must stick to a code of conduct and ethics, and take shared responsibility for the suitability of any product they recommend

****

Chapter 7

Welfare Benefits for Dementia Sufferers, Family and Carers

The benefits system is daunting at the best of times. There are so many benefits available and so many different rules and regulations. However, it is important to gain an understanding of the core benefits that may be available to those who suffer from dementia and those who care for sufferers. As a minimum, a person with dementia can usually claim Attendance Allowance, Disability Living Allowance (care component) or the new Personal Independence Payment (the daily living component). Carers should check their entitlement to Carer's allowance.

The benefits described below are available in England and Wales. Benefits in Northern Ireland and Scotland largely mirror those in England, but there are some differences (such as with Council tax support). People claiming benefits in Scotland and Northern Ireland should contact the Benefit Enquiry Line in Northern Ireland/Scotland (see end of chapter).

This chapter discusses benefits generally. However, for more in-depth advice on the range of benefits available for those suffering from dementia, or their carers, you should go to the Citizens

Advice website or to The Alzheimer's Society. There is a list of useful addresses at the end of this chapter.

How to claim benefits-Qualifying for benefits

To qualify for any benefit, you will have to meet certain conditions. These vary according to the type of benefit. Some benefits depend on you having paid National Insurance contributions over a period of time, some on the amount of your weekly income and savings, and some on the practical effects of a disability.

Where to claim

The Department for Work and Pensions (DWP) is responsible for administering the state pension and benefits.

The system is organised so that:

- benefits relating to people of working age are dealt with by Jobcentre Plus offices
- the State Pension and other benefits relating to people of state-pension age are dealt with by the Pension Service
- disability benefits are dealt with by the Disability Benefits Centre
- Carer's allowance is dealt with by the Carer's Allowance Unit
- in addition, Her Majesty's Revenue and Customs (HMRC) deal with benefits relating to children, as well as tax credits.

Making a claim

You claim benefits either by filling in forms and sending them in the post, or by phoning a contact centre where an adviser will complete the form and send it to you to sign and return. Some benefits can be claimed by completing an online form on the gov.uk website.

Challenging a decision

Most people receive the benefits they are entitled to without a problem. However, if you believe your claim has been incorrectly turned down, or that you have not been awarded the right amount of benefit, you have the right to challenge the decision. Write to the office that made the decision and ask them to revise it. If they do not alter their decision, you may be able to apply to an independent appeal tribunal.

Challenging a decision can be complex, and seeking advice as soon as possible can really help. Ask your local CAB or advice centre, your local authority's welfare rights unit, or the Alzheimer's Society National Dementia Helpline (details in the useful resources section) .

Care and mobility benefits-Attendance Allowance, Disability Living Allowance and Personal Independence Payments

People with dementia, as anyone else, do not automatically qualify for disability benefits - tests are required to determine the level of need. For people who do qualify, these benefits provide extra help to deal with the practical effects of a disability. They are tax free, and do not depend on National Insurance contributions. Payment is not affected by the person's savings or income. A medical assessment may be required. These benefits are paid at different rates, depending on the person's needs. They can be claimed whether the person works or not, and whether they live alone, with their family or with other people.

If your care needs started after the age of 65, or you have not made a claim until then, you should claim Attendance allowance (AA) (see below). This is for help with personal care, not mobility. If you have care and/or mobility needs and are aged under 65, you should claim Personal independence payment (PIP) instead. You must be under 65 when you make your first claim.

It is important to seek advice if you are already claiming one of these benefits and your needs change. If you are already claiming Disability Living Allowance you should be transferred to PIP by 2018. You don't need to initiate the claim for PIP if you are already getting DLA - you will get an invitation to claim. However, if you don't respond to the invitation, your DLA will be stopped. People who receive PIP before they are 65 will be able to stay on it after they reach 65.

The claim forms for PIP and AA are very detailed and lengthy. There are questions about the activities that the person with dementia finds difficult or impossible to carry out, and about their need for care and supervision. You should consider the bad days as well as the good when thinking about the help needed. It is very important to get advice from a professional (including advice centre staff) on filling in the form to make sure you are giving the information that is needed.

Attendance allowance

Personal care needs might include supervision of, or help with, activities such as washing, dressing, eating, going to the toilet, turning over or settling in bed, taking medication, avoiding danger, or attending social or recreational activities. If you have a disabling condition such as dementia and are over 65, you may qualify for AA at one of the following levels:

- Higher rate - if you need frequent help or prompting with personal care like washing or going to the toilet, or continual supervision to avoid danger during the day and also need help with personal care either for a prolonged period or several times during the night, or if you need watching over.

- Lower rate - if you need frequent help or prompting with personal care, or continual supervision throughout the day, or help either for a prolonged period or several times during the night, or if you need watching over.

Personal Independence Payment

PIP has daily living components and (unlike AA) also mobility components. Depending on your situation, you may qualify for either or both. If you have a disabling condition such as dementia and are under 65, you may qualify for the daily living component of PIP at one of the following levels:

- standard rate - if you have a limited ability to carry out daily living activities
- enhanced rate - if you have a severely limited ability to carry out daily living activities. if you have difficulties getting out and about, you may qualify for the mobility component of PIP at one of the following levels:
- standard rate - if you have limited mobility, which can include the ability to plan a journey or manage it unaided (it's not just about the ability to walk).
- enhanced rate - if you have severely limited mobility (as above).

Making a claim consists of two stages: the basic claim and the claimant questionnaire. The basic claim is made by telephone, or in writing by completing a PIP1 form. This is to establish the claim, and to ensure that you are eligible to apply.

Once the basic claim has been successfully made, a claimant questionnaire (PIP2 - How your disability affects you) will be sent to you. This is aimed at gathering more information about how your health condition or impairment affects your day-to-day life. During the basic claim stage, people who may have additional support needs, for example because of a cognitive impairment, should be contacted by the assessment providers to attend a medical assessment.

Disability living allowance

Although this benefit is being phased out for people aged 16-64, some existing claimants may still be re-assessed for it when their claim comes up for review. This is because they live in an area where PIP isn't yet being introduced for existing claimants. If this affects you, you will need to complete the form as you have in the past, referring to your care and mobility needs as they currently are. You will be re-assessed for PIP at a later date.

If you go into a care home or hospital, temporarily or permanently, get advice about how your AA, PIP or DLA might be affected.

Benefits if unable to work

The following are benefits that can be claimed if you are working but are no longer able to work:

Statutory sick pay

This is paid by employers to employees below retirement age, for up to 28 weeks in any one period of sickness. To qualify, you must earn a set amount or more each week before tax and be off work because of sickness. This benefit is paid at a flat rate and is taxable.

Employment and Support Allowance (ESA)

Employment and Support Allowance has two forms - contributory ESA (which replaced Incapacity benefit) and income-related ESA (which replaced Income support claimed on the grounds of incapacity for work). People with Incapacity benefit or Income support on the grounds of incapacity for work are being transferred to Employment and support allowance. You can still receive Income support if you qualify on grounds other than incapacity - see 'Income support' below.

Carers' needs-Carer's allowance

This benefit can be paid to carers who spend at least 35 hours per week looking after someone who is receiving DLA (care component at highest or middle rate), PIP (daily living component at either rate) or Attendance allowance (at either rate). The carer does not have to be related to, or living with, the person they provide care for.

The benefit does not depend on National Insurance contributions, but it is taxable. It gives most carers who are under State pension age a National Insurance credit each week to help protect their State Pension rights.

Carers must be over 16 when they first claim. In some cases, the person being cared for could lose some of their means-tested benefits if Carer's Allowance is paid, so it is important to seek advice before making a claim.

Carers are not eligible for Carer's Allowance if they earn more than a limited amount each week after the deduction of allowable expenses (such as Income tax and pension contributions), if they are in full-time education, or if they are receiving more than a specified amount from certain other pensions or benefits.

People entitled to Carer's Allowance may be entitled to additional amounts in other benefits they are claiming, such as

Income Support or Pension Credit. This may be the case even for those who are entitled to Carer's Allowance but cannot receive the payments because they are already receiving certain other pensions or benefits. That is, if the person qualifies for Carers Allowance but receives an 'overlapping benefit' - where you are eligible for different benefits but can only receive one at any one time. If you are a carer and are unsure about your entitlement, you should seek advice from Carers UK.

Depending on their income, a carer may be able to claim a higher rate of benefit if their spouse or partner is dependent on them financially. If a carer has dependent children, they may also be able to claim Child Tax Credit.

Retirement-The Pension Service

DWP set up the Pension Service to deal with the State pension and other pension-related benefits. If you have reached, or are nearing, State pension age, the Pension Service will write to you and give you a phone number to call for information. Your queries will usually be dealt with over the phone or by post, but the service can arrange for someone to visit you at home, if necessary.

State pension

A State pension is paid to people who reach State pension age if they have made sufficient National insurance contributions. It is taxable. The State pension age for men is currently 65. The State pension age for women born on or before 5 April 1950 is 60. The pension age for men and women is gradually rising so that by 2020 it will be 66. After that it will rise to 68 for both men and women.

People who do not have sufficient contributions may receive a reduced State pension or no pension at all. Under the previous rules, women and widowed people, divorced people, civil partners and same sex spouses who did not have sufficient contributions of their own were able to claim on the contributions of their partner or former partner. From April 2016 this will no longer be possible.

People may also qualify for extra pension for a number of reasons. People over 80 who do not qualify for a State pension or full State Pension may be eligible for an over-80s pension, which does not depend on National Insurance Contributions.

You can claim your pension if you are still working. However, if you want to, you can defer your pension and then draw a higher weekly pension when you do claim it.

If you are entitled to a State Pension, the Pension Service should contact you about four months before you reach State Pension age. If you have not heard anything three months before reaching State Pension age, contact your social security office or the Pension Service claims line.

There is going to be a new State pension from April 2016, but only for people who reach State pension age on or after April 2016. The basic pension will be set at a higher level for these new retirees, but they will need a longer National insurance record of their own, and certain other pension additions will be phased out.

If you are below State pension age but unable to work, you may be able to protect your State Pension rights by getting National insurance contribution credits. These are automatically given to people receiving certain benefits, such as Incapacity Benefit, Employment and Support allowance and Carer's Allowance.

Alternatively, carers who do not receive these benefits may be able to protect their rights through a weekly carers credit to build up their State Pension entitlement. This scheme replaces the Home Responsibilities Protection Scheme and may make a considerable difference to your State pension. Previous protection built up under the Home Responsibilities Protection Scheme will be incorporated into the new system. If you think you may be eligible, seek advice.

Pension credit

If you are unable to claim the State Pension, or it is not enough for you to live on, you may be entitled to claim other benefits, such as Pension Credit. The age at which men and women are eligible to claim Pension Credit will increase in line with the changes in the State Pension age for women (see 'State Pension' above). Pension Credit is a means-tested benefit. It has two parts: Guarantee Credit and Savings Credit. Guarantee Pension Credit works by topping up a person's income if they are on a low income. Savings Credit is extra money for people aged 65 and over who have an income level above the basic retirement pension level, or who have savings or investments. No new claims for Savings Credit will be taken from April 2016, but people who already receive it will continue to do so.

Some people are entitled to both the Guarantee and Savings Credits, while others are entitled to one or the other. People eligible for Pension Credit may also qualify for other benefits such as help with housing costs, and NHS costs.

Help for people on a low income-Income Support

Income Support is a means-tested benefit to help people with basic living expenses who have not reached the qualifying age for Pension Credit and who are not required to be available for work, such as carers. There are strict criteria for people who qualify for Income support.

You may be able to claim Income Support if you have a low income and limited savings, or limited joint savings with a partner. Whether or not you qualify may depend on the number of hours you and any partner work each week. Income support can be paid in full or as a top up to other pensions and income. If you have a partner, you must claim Income support together.

Income Support does not depend on National Insurance contributions, but savings and income (including income from most benefits) will be taken into account. Income from AA, DLA and PIP will be ignored when calculating weekly income, but savings over a certain amount usually mean you cannot receive

Income sSpport. The amount of Income Support paid varies according to age, existing income and savings, and entitlement to any available premiums.

Premiums are awarded to people receiving certain disability benefits and carers receiving the Carer's Allowance, for example, so it is important to seek advice.

If you are a homeowner, you may receive help with mortgage interest payments, interest payments on loans for certain repairs and improvements, ground rent and some service charges. This will depend on the circumstances of those living in your home. You may not qualify for immediate help with your housing costs.

You can no longer claim Income Support if you cannot work because you have a disability or illness. You should claim ESA instead.

Cold weather and winter fuel payments

Cold weather payments are paid if the average temperature in your area falls or is forecast to fall to freezing point or below for seven consecutive days. These payments are made automatically to people receiving some means-tested benefits including Pension credit and Income support.

If you are of eligible age, you will normally qualify for a winter fuel payment to help with the cost of fuel. The age at which people receive a winter fuel payment is rising because it is linked to the State Pension age for women, which is also increasing (see 'State Pension' above).

People over 80 may be eligible for more money. Many people living in care homes are not eligible for this payment. This benefit is not means-tested or taxable, and will not affect any other benefits you are claiming. For more information, or to apply, contact the Winter fuel payment helpline.

Help with housing costs

If you receive Income Support, income-related Employment and Support Allowance, Income-Related Jobseeker's allowance or Guarantee Credit, you may qualify for help with your rent, Council tax and NHS costs. You may also be eligible to apply for help with your rent and Council Tax if you are on a low income, such as low wages or Savings Credit.

Support for mortgage interest

You may get help paying some of your mortgage interest, if you are entitled to Income Support, Income-Related ESA, income-based Jobseeker's Allowance, or Pension Guarantee Credit (and Universal credit when eventually introduced).

Housing benefit

Housing benefit is a benefit to help pay for rent. It is assessed and paid for by local councils. The amount of benefit paid will normally depend on the person's income and savings, and the rent being charged. You may not be eligible for Housing benefit if you have savings over a set amount.

People renting from a private landlord usually have their Housing Benefit limited to what is known as the Local Housing Allowance. Local Housing Allowance rates can be found on local authority websites. In some instances, a room for a carer can be included in the amounts.

Similar provisions now also apply to people of working age only, living in social sector housing. The under-occupancy size criteria (often referred to as the bedroom tax) means that, if it is considered that you have too many bedrooms, the amount of your rent eligible for housing benefit will be cut by 14% (for one bedroom too many) or 25% (for two or more bedrooms too many).

If you live with a partner, only one of you should apply for Housing Benefit. However, your income and savings will be considered jointly and other adults living with you will affect the amount of Housing Benefit you can receive. Housing benefit does not depend on National Insurance Contributions and is tax free. It can be claimed at the same time as Income Support, Income-Based Jobseeker's Allowance, Income-Related ESA or Pension Credit. A claim form for Housing Benefit is included in the application packs for means-tested benefits.If you are not applying for another benefit you can ask the local authority for an application form.

Help with Council Tax
The Council Tax is set by local authorities to pay for the services they provide. The amount of Council Tax support that a person

or couple is eligible for depends on income and savings, and the amount of Council Tax due. People under pension age may be asked to pay a contribution to the tax even if on a low income.

Help with NHS costs-NHS benefits

People receiving Income Support, Income-Based Jobseeker's Allowance, Pension Credit, Working Tax Credit (a payment that you may qualify for if you work but are on a low income) or income-related ESA might receive help with:

- free prescriptions (prescriptions are also free for anyone aged 60 and over)
- free dental treatment from NHS dentists
- free sight tests and vouchers towards the cost of glasses - sight tests are also free for anyone aged 60 and over
- help with hospital travel costs for NHS treatment and free appliances for outpatients or day patients.

NHS hearing aids are prescribed by an NHS consultant to anyone needing them on free loan. They are fitted, serviced and supplied with batteries free of charge.

NHS low income scheme

If you do not receive any of the above benefits but are on a low income and have savings below the limit, you can apply for help towards NHS health costs. The amount of financial help you receive will depend on your savings and income.

You need to complete form HC1, which you can get from Jobcentre Plus offices and NHS hospitals. Some GPs, dentists and opticians may also stock them. If you live in a care home you can apply on a special short form called HC1(SC). Ask the care home manager or a carer for this form or use the HC1 form. For more information on help with NHS costs, see the booklet HC11 Help with health costs, available from any of the above sources or search for 'HC11' on the Department of Health website.

Special notes

Benefits in hospital

Benefits may be affected if either a carer or a person with dementia goes into an NHS hospital for more than a short stay. In this case, it is important to seek advice and inform the local social security office, Jobcentre Plus office, Pension Centre or DWP Disability and Carers Service as appropriate.

Useful organisations for benefits advice

Age UK
Tavis House
1-6 Tavistock Square
London WC1H 9NA
T 0800 169 6565 (advice line)
E contact@ageuk.org.uk
W www.ageuk.org.uk

Wales - Age Cymru

T 08000 223 444 (advice line)

E enquiries@agecymru.org.uk

W www.agecymru.org.uk

Northern Ireland - Age NI

T 0808 808 7575 (advice line)

E info@ageni.org

W www.ageuk.org.uk/northern-ireland

Provides information and advice for older people in the UK.

Carers UK

20 Great Dover Street

London SE1 4LX

T 0808 808 7777 (advice line) Monday -
Friday 10am-4pm

E advice@carersuk.org

W www.carersuk.org

Citizens Advice Bureau (CAB)

Various locations

W www.citizensadvice.org.uk

www.adviceguide.org.uk

(online information resource)

Your local CAB can provide information and advice in confidence or point you in the right direction to further sources of support. Trained CAB advisers can offer information on benefits in a way that is easy to understand. To find your nearest

CAB, look in the phone book, ask at your local library or look on the website (above). Opening times vary.

Department of Health
Richmond House
79 Whitehall
London SW1A 2NS
T 020 7210 4850 (8.30am-5.30pm weekdays)
020 7210 5025 (textphone)
E use the enquiry form on the website (see below)
W www.dh.gov.uk

The government department responsible for health, social care, and the National Health Service (NHS). Provides a range of information and literature, including help with NHS costs.

Department for Work and Pensions (DWP)
W www.gov.uk
The government department responsible for employment and social security. The gov.uk website gives details of the various benefits and how to claim them, as well as information on pensions and pension credits. Claim forms are available to download.

Disability Benefits Centre
W www.gov.uk/disability-benefits-helpline

Personal Independence Payment (PIP)
T 0345 850 3322

Textphone: 0345 601 6677
Monday to Friday, 8am-6pm

Personal Independence Payment
(New claims only)
T 0800 917 2222
Textphone: 0800 917 7777
Monday to Friday, 8am-6pm

Disability Living Allowance
T 0345 712 3456
Textphone: 0345 722 4433
Monday to Friday, 8am-6pm

Attendance Allowance (also for DLA claimants who are 65+)
T 0345 605 6055
Textphone: 0345 604 5312
Monday to Friday, 8am-6pm

Winter Fuel Payments Helpline
T 0845 915 1515 (8.30am-4.30pm weekdays)
W www.gov.uk/winter-fuel-payment

State Pension and Pension Credit enquiries
T 0345 60 60 265 (8am-6pm weekdays)
State pension claim line
T 0800 731 7898 (8am-6pm weekdays)
W www.gov.uk/state-pension

NHS Help with health costs advice line
T 0300 330 1343
Provides NHS patients with information about entitlements to prescription charge exemptions and the requirements to qualify for exemptions.

Northern Ireland - Benefit Enquiry Line
T 0800 220 674 (9am-5pm weekdays except
Thursday; 10am-5pm Thursday)
028 9031 1092 (textphone, 9am-5pm weekdays)

Provides advice and information on Attendance allowance, Disability living allowance, Personal independence payments, Carer's allowance and Carer's credit.

Welfare benefits Scotland
https://www.citizensadvice.org.uk/scotland/benefits

****

Chapter 8

The importance of Diet and Exercise in the Control of Dementia

---

Dementia and Exercise

So far in this book, we have discussed areas of a practical nature which will help guide a person or their carer through dealing with Dementia. Two very important areas, which we have decided to leave to the last, are those of exercise and diet.

We fully realise that whilst you are trying to cope with all of the other effects of Dementia, the importance of exercise and diet may be low on your list of considerations. However, they are areas of great importance in the overall plan of helping a person with dementia to maintain a healthy life and maintain good health generally.

Sadly, it is recognized that there are those in advanced states of Dementia who cannot manage to exercise regularly, if at all. However, whilst you can, or whilst the sufferer perhaps can still undertake some exercise, it is essential to have a daily regime. In order to ensure that you are doing all you can to stay fit and healthy, great care must be taken to ensure that you are in good shape and eat well. This acts as a kind of insurance policy against the encroachments of Dementia. In addition, people are also encouraged to exercise regularly to reduce the risk of cardiovascular diseases.

Additional benefits of exercise include a healthier heart, better weight control and stress management all of which are essential to maintain mental and physical health.

The Importance of exercise

As well as strengthening the cardiovascular system and the body's muscles, many people exercise to keep fit, lose or maintain a healthy weight, sharpen their athletic skills, or purely for enjoyment. Regular, frequent physical exercise is recommended for people of all age groups as it boosts the immune system and helps to protect against conditions such as:

- Heart disease
- Stroke
- Type 2 diabetes
- Cancer and other major illnesses

In fact, it is known to cut your risk of major chronic illnesses/diseases by up to 50% and reduce your risk of early death by up to 30%. There are other health benefits of exercising on a regular basis which include:

- Improvements in mental health
- It boosts self-esteem/confidence
- It enhances sleep quality and energy levels
- It cuts risk of stress and depression

- Very importantly, it protects against Dementia and Alzheimer's disease

Defining exercise

In the UK, regular exercise is defined by the NHS as completing 150 minutes of moderate intensity aerobic activity a week. Aerobic activity at moderate intensity means exercising at a level that raises your heart rate and makes you sweat. This includes a multitude of sports. For example;

- Walking at a fast pace
- Jogging lightly
- Bike riding
- Rowing
- Playing tennis or badminton
- Water aerobics

The less time you spend sitting down, the better it will be for your health. Sedentary behaviour, such as sitting or lying down for long periods, increases your risk of weight gain and obesity, which in turn, may also up your risk of chronic diseases such as heart disease.

Dementia and diet

It is a fact that eating well is important, whether or not a person has dementia. The foods you choose to eat in your daily diet make a difference to how well you feel and how much energy you have every day. How much you need to eat and drink is based on your age, gender, how active you are and the goals you are looking to achieve.

Portion sizes have grown in recent years, as the plates and bowls we use have got bigger. Use smaller crockery to cut back on your portion sizes, while making the food on your plate look bigger. No single food contains all the essential nutrients you need in the right proportion. That's why you need to consume foods from each of the main food groups to eat well.

Fruit and vegetables

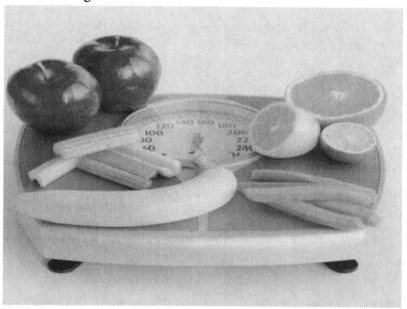

Naturally low in fat and calories and packed full of vitamins, minerals and fibre, fruit and vegetables add flavour and variety to every meal. They may also help protect against stroke, heart disease, high blood pressure and some cancers. Everyone should eat at least five portions a day. Fresh, frozen, dried and canned fruit in juice and canned vegetables in water all count. Go for a rainbow of colours to get as wide a range of vitamins and minerals as possible. Try:

- adding an apple, banana, pear, or orange with your lunch
- sliced melon or grapefruit topped with low-fat yogurt, or a handful of berries, or fresh dates, apricots or prunes for breakfast
- carrots, peas and green beans mixed up in a pasta bake
- adding an extra handful of vegetables to your dishes when cooking – peas to rice, spinach to lamb or onions to chicken.

Starchy foods

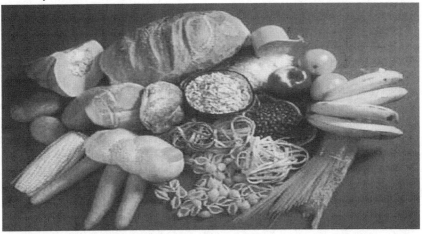

Potatoes, rice, pasta, bread, chapattis, naan and plantain all contain carbohydrate, which is broken down into glucose and used by your cells as fuel.

Better options of starchy foods – such as wholegrain bread, wholewheat pasta and basmati, brown or wild rice – contain more fibre, which helps to keep your digestive system working well. They are generally more slowly absorbed (that is, they have a lower glycaemic index, or GI), keeping you feeling fuller for longer. Try to include some starchy foods every day.

Try:

- two slices of multigrain toast with a scraping of spread and Marmite or peanut butter or stir-fries
- potatoes any way you like – but don't fry them – with the skin left on for valuable fibre. Choose low-fat toppings, such as cottage cheese or beans
- baked sweet potato, with the skin left on for added fibre
- boiled cassava, flavoured with chilli and lemon
- chapatti made with brown or wholemeal atta.

Meat, fish, eggs, pulses, beans and nuts

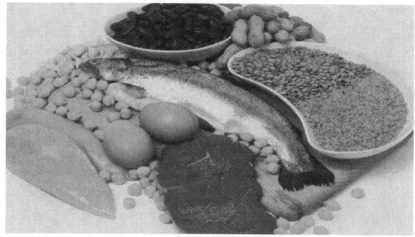

These foods are high in protein, which helps with building and replacing muscles. They contain minerals, such as iron, which are vital for producing red blood cells. Oily fish, such as mackerel, salmon and sardines, also provide omega-3, which can help protect the heart. Beans, pulses, soya and tofu are also good sources of protein. Aim to have some food from this group every day, with at least 1–2 portions of oily fish a week. Try:

- serving meat, poultry or a vegetarian alternative grilled, roasted or stir-fried
- a small handful of raw nuts and seeds as a snack or chopped with a green salad
- using beans and pulses in a casserole to replace some – or all – of the meat
- grilled fish with masala, fish pie, or make your own fish cakes
- eggs scrambled, poached, dry fried or boiled – the choice is yours!

Dairy foods

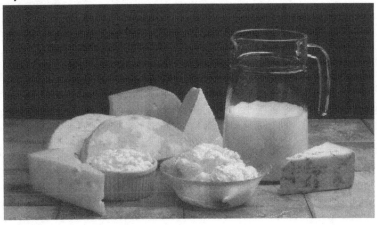

Milk, cheese and yogurt contain calcium, which is vital to keep bones and teeth strong. They're good sources of protein, too.

Some dairy foods are high in fat, particularly saturated fat, so choose lower-fat alternatives (check for added sugar, though). Semi-skimmed milk actually contains more calcium than whole milk, but children under 2 should have whole milk because they may not get the calories or essential vitamins they need from lower-fat milks. Try:

- milk straight in a glass, flavoured with a little cinnamon, or added to breakfast porridge
- yogurt with fruit or on curry
- cottage cheese scooped on carrot sticks
- a bowl of breakfast cereal in the morning, with skimmed or semi-skimmed milk
- a cheese sandwich at lunchtime, packed with salad
- a refreshing lassi or some plain yogurt with your evening meal.

Foods high in fat and sugar

You can enjoy food from this group as an occasional treat in a balanced diet, but remember that sugary foods and drinks will add extra calories – and sugary drinks will raise blood glucose – so opt for diet/light or low-calorie alternatives. Or choose water – it's calorie free!

Fat is high in calories, so try to reduce the amount of oil or butter you use in cooking. Remember to use unsaturated oils, such as sunflower, rapeseed or olive oil, as these types are better for your heart.

Salt

Too much salt can make you more at risk of high blood pressure and stroke. Processed foods can be very high in salt. Try cooking more meals from scratch at home, where you can control the amount of salt you use – when there are so many delicious spices in your kitchen, you really can enjoy your favourite recipes with less salt.

Adults should have no more than 1 tsp (6g) of salt a day, while children have even lower targets.

Try:

- banishing the salt cellar from the table, but keeping the black pepper.
- seasoning food with herbs and spices, instead of salt. Try ginger, lime and coriander in stir-fries, or use spicy harissa paste to flavour soups, pasta dishes and couscous.
- making fresh chutney using coriander leaves (dhaniya), fresh mint, chopped green chillies and lime juice.
- measuring added salt in cooking with a teaspoon and use less as time goes on. Do it gradually, and the family will hardly notice!
- flavouring salads with lemon juice, chilli powder and pepper.

- making your own tandoori marinade in seconds using red chilli powder, ground garam masala, paprika powder, low-fat plain yogurt, garlic, ginger, and tomato purée.
- adding finely chopped coriander leaves to lassi, and sprinkle on ground jeera and ground coriander seeds.

Combined together, diet and exercise can prove invaluable in helping to combat dementia, and will also contribute to a persons well-being if dementia has already set in.

****

Useful addresses and contacts

The following , although not exhaustive, is a list of organisations and their websites and contact details.

Dementia-general organisations

Action on Elder Abuse enquiries@elderabuse.org.uk
www.elderabuse.org.uk

Advice UK www.adviceuk.org.uk
This is an online hub signposting to organisations advising on benefits, legal matters, financial and other issues.

AGE UK advice line www.ageuk.org.uk
0800 169 2081, provides information about help available through social services, as well as advice about other issues faced by older people. Local services can include: information, advice and advocacy services; day centres and lunch clubs; home help and 'handyperson' schemes; and IT and other training.

Wales - Age Cymru
T 0800 169 6565
E enquiries@agecymru.org.uk
W http://www.agecymru.org.uk/

Northern Ireland - Age NI W www.ageuk.org.uk/northern-ireland

T 0808 808 7575

E info@ageni.org

Alzheimer's Research UK

0300 111 5555

www.alzheimersresearch.org

Alzheimer's Society www.alzheimers.co.uk

The Alzheimer's Society Provides the National Dementia Helpline in England, Wales and Northern Ireland on 0300 222 1122. It offers information, support, guidance and signposting to other appropriate organisations.

Alzheimer Scotland www.alzscot.org

Alzheimer Scotland provides the National Dementia Helpline 0808 808 3000 in Scotland as well as local services all over Scotland for people with dementia and their carers.

AT Dementia www.atdementia.org.uk

AT Dementia Provides information about assistive technology for people with dementia. Assistive technology can be any device or system that helps someone perform a task. This includes devices like calendar clocks, automatic lighting and fall sensors.

Citizens Advice Bureau (CAB)

Various locations

W http://www.citizensadvice.org.uk/

http://www.adviceguide.org.uk/

Your local CAB can provide information and advice in confidence or point you in the right direction. To find your nearest CAB look in the phone book, ask at your local library or look on the Citizens Advice website (above). Opening times vary.

Civil Legal Advice W www.gov.uk/civil-legal-advice
T 08453 454 345 (9am-8pm weekdays, 9am-12.30pm Saturday)

Provides free and confidential legal advice in England and Wales if you're eligible for legal aid.

Court of Protection
PO Box 70185
First Avenue House
42-49 High Holborn
London WC1A 9JA
T 0300 456 4600
E courtofprotectionenquiries@hmcts.gsi.gov.uk
W www.gov.uk/apply-to-the-court-of-protection

The Court of Protection makes decisions and appoints deputies to act on behalf of people who are unable to make decisions about their personal health, finance or welfare.

Dementia NI www.alzheimers.org.uk/northernireland
Dementia NI Campaigns to raise awareness of dementia and provides training and education on living well with the condition. It has groups around Northern Ireland helping people with dementia to meet and support each other.

Dementia UK www.dementia.uk.org

Dementia UK provides mental health nurses who specialise in dementia, called Admiral Nurses. They provide practical and emotional support to families affected by dementia. They can also provide advice on referrals to appropriate services and liaise with other healthcare professionals on your behalf. To find out if Admiral Nurses are available in your area, you can call their helpline – 0800 888 6678.

Disabled Living Foundation
Ground Floor, Landmark House
Hammersmith Bridge Road
London W6 9EJ
T 0845 130 9177 (helpline 10am-4pm weekdays)
E info@dlf.org.uk
W www.dlf.org.uk

Charity that provides information about finding simple solutions, such as mobility aids. Offers a loan library of simple electronic aids that people in England can borrow for two weeks to see if they work. (See www.dlf.org.uk/library)

Foundation for Assistive Technology (FAST)
302 Tower Bridge Business Centre
46-48 East Smithfield
London E1W 1AWT 0300 330 1430
E info@fastuk.org
W www.fastuk.org

Charity that works with the assistive technology community to get well-designed, useful inventions on to the market faster. Provides an online database of assistive technology research, events and contacts.

Guideposts www.guideposts.org

Guideposts provides services for people with long-term or degenerative conditions, including dementia. They also provide an online and telephone information resource called HERE which helps people to find out about support and care services. Call 0300 222 5709.

Independent Age www.independentage.org

Independent Age provides information and advice for older people, their families and carers. They focus on social care, welfare benefits and befriending services. The helpline can give advice on home care, care homes, NHS services and housing. Their helpline number is 0800 319 6789.

Law Society

113 Chancery Lane

London WC2A 1PL

T 020 7242 1222 (general enquiries)

 020 7320 5650 (for help finding a solicitor)

E findasolicitor@lawsociety.org.uk

W http://www.lawsociety.org.uk/

The body representing solicitors in England and Wales. It provides details of law firms and solicitors practising in England and Wales, and useful information about legal specialities and fees, as well as tips about what to ask and what to expect from a solicitor.

MIND
www.mind.org
0300123 3393
Mental health Charity that publishes information on all aspects of mental health and provides a range of support through local associations.

NHS Choices www.nhs.uk
www.nhs.uk/service-search (for local services)
www.nhs.uk/carersdirect or call 0808 802 0202
The UK's biggest health website provides a comprehensive health information service that aims to put people in control of their healthcare.

NHS Direct Wales
www.nhsdirect.wales.nhs.uk 0845 4647

Solicitors for the Elderly
Mill Studio Business Centre
Crane Mead
Ware
Hertfordshire SG12 9PY
T 0844 567 6173
E admin@solicitorsfortheelderly.com
W www.solicitorsfortheelderly.com

Independent, national organisation of lawyers who provide legal advice to older people. They can also help you to find a solicitor.

The British Red Cross www.RedCross.org.uk
The British Red Cross can help people following a short stay in hospital by providing extra support and care at home. Call 0344 871 11 11.

The Office of the Public Guardian
www.gov.uk/.../organisations/office-of-the-public-guardian
They can be contacted on 0300 456 0300 for information and advice about Lasting Power of Attorney.

The Wales Dementia Helpline www.nhsdirect.wales.nhs.uk
Wales Dementia Offers help and support to people with dementia in Wales, their carers, family members or friends. Their helpline number is 0808 808 2235.

RADAR - the Disability Rights People
Disability Rights UK
12 City Forum
250 City Road
London EC1V 8AF
T 020 7250 3222
E enquiries@disabilityrightsuk.org
W www.radar-shop.org.uk

The RADAR National Key Scheme offers disabled people independent access to locked public toilets around the country.

Toilets fitted with National Key Scheme locks can now be found in shopping centres, pubs, cafés, department stores, bus and train stations and many other locations in most parts of the country.

UK Homecare Association Ltd
www.ukhca.co.uk 020 8661 8188
The national association for organisations who provide social care, including nursing services for people in their own homes.

Rare Dementia Support www.raredementiasupport.org
Rare Dementia Support runs specialist support services for people living with, or affected by, five rare dementias: frontotemporal dementia (FTD), posterior cortical atrophy (PCA), primary progressive aphasia (PPA), familial Alzheimer's disease (FAD) and familial frontotemporal dementia (fFTD). They provide regular support group meetings, newsletters, telephone contact networks and access to information and advice..

The Lewy Body Society and Parkinson's UK lewybody.org
www.parkinsons.org.uk

Both of the Societies provide support and information about dementia with Lewy bodies (DLB). As well as supporting people with Parkinson's disease, Parkinson's UK can also help with questions about Parkinson's dementia. The helpline service for both is provided by Parkinson's UK. You can contact a helpline advisor on 0808 800 0303.

The PSP Association www.pspassociation.org.uk
The PSP Association helps people with progressive supranuclear palsy (PSP) and corticobasal degeneration (CBD). It offers advice, support and information to people living with these conditions. You can call their helpline on 0300 0110 122.

Young Dementia UK www.youngdementiauk.org
YoungDementia UK provides information, advice and support for people under 65 diagnosed with dementia, their family and friends. General enquiries 01993 776295

Organisations for people with bladder and bowel problems

Bladder and Bowel Foundation
SATRA Innovation Park
Rockingham Road
Kettering NN16 9JH
T 01536 533255 (general enquiries)
0845 345 0165 (helpline)
E info@bladderandbowelfoundation.org
W www.bladderandbowelfoundation.org

A charity for adults affected by bladder and bowel problems. It provides information and support for individuals, patients, carers and healthcare professionals. The Foundation also sells the Just Can't Wait toilet card.

PromoCon
Disabled Living
Burrows House
10 Priestley Road
Wardley Industrial Estate
Worsley
Manchester M28 2LY
T 0161 607 8219
E promocon@disabledliving.co.uk
W www.disabledliving.co.uk/promocon/about

Provides a national service to improve life for all people with bladder or bowel problems by offering product information, advice and practical solutions to professionals and the general public.

Organisations for carers

Babble (Carers Trust online community for carers under 18) Young carers hub (NHS Choices)

Carers Direct www.carersdirect.com
Carers Direct provides a national helpline service for carers, offering confidential information and advice. This service is part of the NHS and can be contacted on 0300 123 1053. A webchat is available on the website.

Carers UK www.carersuk.org

Carers UK provides advice and information to carers. This is available through the website, booklets, factsheets and their Adviceline 70808 808 777.

Care Information Scotland www.careinfoscotland.co.uk
Care Information Scotland is a telephone and website service. They provide information about care services for older people in Scotland. This service is funded by the Scottish government and run by NHS 24. Their helpline number is 0800 011 3200.

The Carers Trust carers.org
The Carers Trust works to improve support, services and recognition for anyone living with the challenges of caring, unpaid, for a family member or friend who is ill, frail, disabled or has mental health or addiction problems. Call 0844 800 4361.

Young carers (Barnardos) www.barnardos.org.uk

Accommodation, housing and care homes

The Elderly Accommodation Counsel www.eac.org.uk
The Elderley Accommodation Counsel helps older people make choices about housing and care. They run FirstStop Advice. This telephone service, on 0800 377 7070, offers advice and information to older people, their families and carers about housing and care options.

Commercial care providers

There are a large number of providers of care and social services..
A good place to start looking for services is the Care Quality
Commission. You can search for local care services on their
website www.cqc.org.uk. Call them on 03000 616 161.

Holidays for people with dementia and their carers

Amy's Care
Nestled in the middle of a traditional Cumbrian fell village, near
Keswick, Amy's Holiday's has developed a beautiful holiday
home complete with disabled facilities which is available to hire
with, or without, care. With fully qualified staff available to
attend the property to help with any care needed and day care
already offered within the village Amy's can facilitate a holiday
for all the family.
http://www.amys-care.co.uk/
Telephone: 016973 71087
Email rebecca@amys-care.co.uk
Telephone: 01457 833 444.

Cherish Dementia Holiday Trust
120 Ridge Lane
Nuneaton
CV10 0RD
Telephone: 01827 768569
E-mail: cherish-dementia-trust@hotmail.com

The aim of Cherish Dementia Holidays is to provide assisted holidays and day trips to people with Dementia and their Carers, usually husbands or wives, daughters or sons or anyone who provides a substantial amount of care. Importantly each couple needs to be self-caring as no personal care is on offer.

Specifically the organisation:-

- Provides short holidays and day trips for those with dementia and their carers
- Encourages social inclusion by bringing together people with care responsibilities from all sections of the community for mutual support
- Gives those caring for people with dementia the ability to take a rewarding holiday with support to care for their loved ones
- Provides opportunities for carers and those people being cared for to experience a different environment giving them a break from their day-to-day routine
- Manages the holiday experience and makes holiday arrangements on behalf of the carer and person cared for ensuring they are free to enjoy their holiday without the responsibility of arranging it.

Dementia Adventure

Dementia Adventure is a social enterprise specialising in connecting people living with dementia with nature and a sense of adventure. They focus on the individual aiming to relieve the needs of people living with dementia and their carers by

providing or assisting in the provision of holidays, outdoor activities and other support.
www.dementiaadventure.co.uk
Tel: 01245 237548
Email: info@dementiaadventure.co.uk

Disabled Holidays
www. disabledholidays.com/about/alzheimer's/travel tips

Disabled Holidays is a travel agency which arranges holidays for people with disabilities, illnesses and medical conditions and for people with limited or no mobility. They can arrange end of life holidays with diligence and dignity. They have accommodation that is accessible and suitable for your needs. they also arrange for the hiring of any equipment you might require.

MindforYou
MindforYou provides supported holidays, for people living with dementia and their carers. Our small groups of up to 14 likeminded people and our high staff ratio give you a personalised break. We identify dementia friendly properties and use assistive technologies, to ensure you both enjoy your holiday together with MindforYou.
www.mindforyou.co.uk
Tel: 07788 292 938
Email: info@mindforyou.co.uk

Revitalise
Revitalise is a national charity offering a wide range of accessible breaks for disabled adults and carers. The essence of all their breaks is freedom and choice.

Throughout the year they offer a number of weeks specifically for guests with Alzheimer's and other types of dementia, and their partners or carers.

They make sure that partners and carers get some time to themselves with the assurance that their staff are on hand at all times to support you and your loved ones. Because they provide the care you can enjoy spending some quality time together too.

Revitalise subsidises the cost of all their Alzheimer's breaks so they are able to offer guests reduced prices.

For more information on any of their services visit their website http://revitalise.org.uk/.
Tel: 0303 303 0145
Email: bookings@revitalise.org.uk

End of life care

Cruse Bereavement Care www.cruse.org.uk
CRUSE offers support, advice and information to people when someone dies, through their freephone national helpline, 0808 808 1677. They also provide training for those who may encounter bereaved people in the course of their work. They have a website specifically for children and young people.

Dying Matters
T 0800 021 4466
W www.dyingmatters.org
www.dyingmatters.org/contact (web form)

Dying Matters is a broad-based and inclusive national coalition led by the National Council for Palliative Care. It aims to change public knowledge, attitudes and behaviours towards dying, death and bereavement. They produce information to help people talk about death, dying and bereavement, including a 'Preferred priorities for care' form to complete. You can search for local services via the website.

National Council for Palliative Care (NCPC)
The Fitzpatrick Building
188–194 York Way
London N7 9AS
T 020 7697 1520
E enquiries@ncpc.org.uk
W www.ncpc.org.uk

The National Council for Palliative Care (NCPC) is the umbrella charity for all those involved in palliative, end-of-life and hospice care in England, Wales and Northern Ireland. They work with government, health and social care staff and people with personal experience to improve end-of-life care for all. They also produce information to help people talk about death and dying.

****

Index

Jogging, 111
Joint-accounts, 5, 63

Lasting powers of Attorney, 4, 58
Lewy body dementia, 3, 17, 21, 22
Long-term physical disability, 67

Meat, 114
Medicines, 36
Memantine hydrochloride, 28
Memory loss, 21, 22
Mental Capacity Act 2005, 75
Multi-infarct dementia, 21

National Institute for Health and Care Excellence (NICE, 30
Neurons, 19
NHS, 111
NHS continuing healthcare, 6, 69, 83, 84

Occupational therapist, 34
Omega-3, 115
Outdoor safety., 40

Parkinson's disease, 3, 17, 18, 24, 126
Post-stroke dementia, 21
Potatoes, 113
Processed foods, 117
Professional support, 4, 45
Property and affairs deputyship, 4, 57
Protein, 115, 116
Psychological treatments, 3, 29
Pulses, 114, 115

****

Other titles in the Emerald Series

Emerald
www.straightfowardpublishing.co.uk

Titles in the Emerald Series:

Law
Guide to Bankruptcy
Conducting Your Own Court case
Creating a Will
Guide to European Union Law
Guide to Health and Safety Law
Guide to Criminal Law
Guide to Landlord and Tenant Law
Guide to the English Legal System
Guide to Housing Law
Guide to Marriage and Divorce
Guide to The Civil Partnerships Act
The Path to Justice
You and Your Legal Rights
Powers of Attorney
Managing Divorce

Health
Guide to Combating Child Obesity
Asthma Begins at Home
Alternative Health and Alternative Remedie

General
A Practical Guide to Obtaining probate
A Practical Guide to Residential Conveyancing

Keeping Books and Accounts-A Small Business Guide
Business Start Up-A Guide for New Business
Finding Asperger Syndrome in the Family-A Book of Answers
Explaining Autism Spectrum Disorder
Explaining Alzheimers
Explaining Parkinsons
Writing True Crime
Becoming a Professional Writer
Writing your Autobiography
Self-hypnosis
Waiting for a Voice-Guide to Verbal Dyspraxia

For details of the above titles published by Emerald go to:

www.straightforwardpublishing.co.uk